Constructing
the Erotic

Constructing
the Erotic

Sexual Ethics and
Adolescent Girls

BARBARA J. BLODGETT

THE
PILGRIM
PRESS
Cleveland

The Pilgrim Press, 700 Prospect Avenue, Cleveland, Ohio 44115-1100
pilgrimpress.com

08   07   06   05   04   03   02   5   4   3   2   1

Library of Congress Cataloging-in-Publication Data
Blodgett, Barbara J., 1961-
    Constructing the erotic : sexual ethics and adolescent girls / Barbara J.
Blodgett.
      p. cm.
    ISBN 0-8298-1478-7
    1. Sex instruction for girls. 2. Sexual ethics for teenagers.   I. Title.
HQ51 .B56 2002
613.9′55 – dc21

                              2002016951

Contents

Preface

THE CHRISTIAN FEMINIST COMMUNITY, in which I include myself, has made significant contributions to sexual ethics by insisting that human sexuality is a good gift of God's creation. This book nevertheless critiques a group of feminist theologians and ethicists whose faith in a new vision of human sexuality I consider premature. These "feminist theologies of the erotic," as I call them, represent a movement to recover the classic notion of the erotic as a drive toward fullness of life, to reinterpret this concept as a feminist one, and to proclaim the erotic a liberating resource and moral guide. I laud their work but judge it ultimately unsuccessful. Rather than a sexual ethic based on the erotic, I recommend a sexual ethic based on establishing appropriate vulnerability and trust. Such an ethic is ultimately more helpful, especially for adolescent girls whose experience of the erotic is frequently not liberating.

After an introductory chapter, the book explores feminist theologies of the erotic and engages in a critique of five feminist theologians — Audre Lorde, Carter Heyward, Rita Nakashima Brock, Anne Bathurst Gilson, and Marvin Ellison. In chapter 3, I place their work in historical context and read it as a response to earlier, liberal feminist theology. I identify some necessary correctives, including especially the need for a social constructionist framework to alleviate universalizing tendencies.

Chapter 4 then examines empirical evidence of erotic experience from adolescent girls' narratives about sex and romance. Comparison reveals that feminist theologians of the erotic are overly confident about the possibilities for erotic liberation. Girls are constrained by their gender. Their self-disavowal and preoccupation with romance render any simple naming and claiming of erotic experience impossible. In chapter 5, I use feminist psychological and psychoanalytic theories to interpret the empirical evidence and to explain how girls' erotic experience is constructed starting early in life. This perspective underscores the complexity of the erotic and the need to theorize it as a construct of power relations. Finally, in chapter 6, I propose that a discourse of sexual ethics must be one of vulnerability and trust rather than Eros and liberation. Examining the phenomenon of interpersonal trust, and drawing upon philosophical literature as well as debates about trust within professional ethics, I apply an ethic of trust to a sexual ethic for adolescents.

This book began as my Ph.D. dissertation at Yale University. At the beginning, when I was in the process of choosing a dissertation topic, some graduate students in my program were electing to write on the classic themes of theological ethics, while others were choosing to address the groundbreaking ethical questions of the day. In contrast, I knew that I wanted to consider something relatively ordinary yet important to the lives of contemporary women like myself, and thus arose my decision to write about the ethics of sex. Then I formed a dissertation writing group composed of women from several different departments who were writing on feminist topics. At our inaugural meeting we told each other why we had chosen to write on our topics. That gathering was the first of many experiences I would have of explaining to people that writing about sex was not nearly as exciting as it sounded! The topic grew only more interesting, however, during the years it took to complete the project.

I have many people to thank for supporting me and thinking with me throughout this project: my family, my teachers and mentors at Yale — Serene Jones, Tom Ogletree, Gene Outka, and especially Margaret Farley — my colleagues and students in the Department of Religion at Oberlin College, and my editor at The Pilgrim Press, George Graham, who has been so enthusiastic. I want to thank especially my friends Brian Stiltner and Stephen Edmondson, who read portions of the manuscript, and Kaudie McLean, who edited it. Above all, I thank the members of my writing group, without whom this book could not have been written: Kathleen Clark, Alexa Freeman, Jane Levey, Jennifer Manion, Rachel Roth, and Eve Weinbaum.

ONE

Acknowledging
the Complex Meanings
of Sexual Experience

> Why sexuality, rather than love? Is not love the comprehensive term, the ascendant pole, the spiritual motivation? Certainly. But sexuality is the domain of all the difficulties, all the gropings, the dangers and the dilemmas, the failure and the joy. — Paul Ricoeur, "Wonder, Eroticism, and Enigma"

B EING TOO CONFIDENT about the true meaning of human sexual experience is imprudent. Even more imprudent is to claim that once the true meaning of human sexual experience is known, the truth will set us free. Consider three stories.

Kathleen Sands tells the story of attending a session of the American Academy of Religion in 1990 on "Exploring the Links between Sexual Experience and Women's Religious Lives." Most of the presenters offered positive renderings of sexual experience as a resource for women's liberation and flourishing. But one of the papers included a harrowing account of sexual abuse and its devastating effect on young girls' spirits. Sands recalls how palpable the irony was:

> Afterwards, the room fell quiet, silenced by the encounter with brutal experience. Finally, someone spoke, raising what has become for me the most difficult question feminist theology faces in regard to sex: How could [these] painful insights be reconciled with the other presenters' positive views of Eros? Two presenters hastened to offer what seems to have become a standard response in feminist theology. Sexual abuse of any kind, they said, is not Eros; in fact, it is the opposite of Eros. I agree, of course, that sexual abuse is the opposite of *ideal* Eros. Who could disagree? But the speakers seemed to be

1

saying more than that. Their claims for Eros sounded more like articles of a transcendent faith than actual responses to the experiential
agony of incest.[1]

The second story, though less dramatic, pinpoints a similar frustration
with current theological thinking about Eros. I attended a session of the
Society of Christian Ethics several years ago to hear a prominent ethicist
deliver a paper on the social construction of human sexual desire.[2] Christian ethicists are sometimes loath to embrace social constructionism out
of a fear that if the meaning of something is always shifting, judging it
right or wrong is impossible. This presenter, however, was arguing that
Christian ethicists should resist the urge to reduce the meaning of sexual
desire to a single purpose, and they should especially avoid reducing such
desire to a purely biological explanation, as sociobiologists would do. Instead, he said, we should affirm a multiplicity of meanings behind human
sexual desire and seek their genesis in the social environment. Sexual desire, like other human feelings and emotions, he argued, is not a mere
reflex or involuntary response to stimuli, but rather a passion evoked and
shaped by our cognitive understanding of what will be fulfilling. Our
understanding of what will be fulfilling is, in turn, reflective of our social
environment and its worlds of meaning. In other words, sexual desire is
to a large extent socially constructed. At the same time, he did not want
to relinquish the notion that human sexual desire is also to some extent
determined by basic biological needs — that we just want certain things
sexually because our nature is to want them. In the end, his compromise
(the details of which need not concern us here) was to affirm that physical,
biologically driven urges for sex exist in reciprocal relationship to social
desires. For example, seeking sexual union with a mate goes hand in hand
with a yearning for intimacy constructed by social understandings of fulfillment and love. An impulse to pleasure one's partner correlates with
a desire to share affection in mutual relationship. An inclination toward
sexual demonstrativeness corresponds to flirting, and so on. The presenter
wished to argue, in effect, that our biologically driven desires line up in
neat correspondence to the erotic desires to which we are socialized.

---

1. Kathleen Sands, "Uses of the Thea(o)logian: Sex and Theodicy in Religious Feminism,"
Journal for the Feminist Study of Religion 8 (spring 1992): 7.
2. Timothy Sedgwick, paper delivered at the Society of Christian Ethics Annual Meeting,
February 1993.

But all of his examples were of positive, healthy eroticism. They did not admit of an unseemly side to sex. They did not address whether a biological impulse may exist behind someone's desire to bully, tease, or conquer another person sexually. Consequently, these examples raised the following question: Must not the meaning of "sexual desire" be expansive enough to include, say, a desire to dominate another person sexually as well as a desire to unite with them in love? The implication is that, if so, ethicists would have to bring the biological determinism/social constructionism debate to bear on such a desire as well and make some sense of it. During the period for discussion following the talk, I asked that very question. The presenter dismissed my inquiry. His response was flatly to say that clearly the type of "desire" I had named was wrong, his implication being that we did not need to make any sense of that desire because it was a perversity. This response disappointed me, the way Kathleen Sands had felt disappointed. Of course I agree that sexual domination is wrong, but that does not make the desire to dominate go away; what's more, as Christian ethicists who embrace a plurality of meanings of sexuality, we cannot ignore possible meanings that strike us as perverse and make us uncomfortable. If we ignore them, we offer no practical help to those Christians (perhaps not a tiny minority) who experience the "wrong" desires.

A final example comes from feminist social historian Sharon Thompson, who chronicles teenage girls' experiences of romance, sex, and love. Thompson says that feminists who strive to change the social conditions under which the next generation comes of age often alienate girls by telling them only about the evils and dangers of sexual activity in a patriarchal world. Girls, she argues, also need to hear of the potential pleasures of sexuality and romance, if only because pleasure might characterize at least part of their experience, even under patriarchy. Girls furthermore deserve to be able to make sense of the exciting pull that romance exerts on them, as well as the pain it can and often does cause. Thompson writes:

> One wing of the feminist movement talks solely in terms of rape, incest, molestation, and exploitation. There is unquestionably a place in feminism for this work. But in not acknowledging the limits of a politics that deals with only sexual violence and not with other sexual and romantic themes, and in conflating violence with sexuality, this work often fails to describe, or leave space for, the breadth of teenage girls' experience. . . . Effective feminist work with teenagers

must speak to the magnetism and concerns of sex and romance, not dismiss them.[3]

These stories demonstrate the multiple dangers in overconfidence about the meaning of Eros or sexuality. The first shows how feminist theologians work themselves into a trap by their own exuberance about the value of erotic experience to human flourishing. The second shows that even someone who wishes to affirm that sexual desires are not merely "given" but also socially constructed can nevertheless discount psychological urges that are socially unacceptable. The third shows that preconceptions about the gender politics of sexuality can blind feminists to the ways women have survived and even thrived despite oppression. All three stories are ironic, for the reformers falter precisely in trying to reform inherited understandings of sexuality. The irony magnifies because hearing Christian theologians and feminists like these speaking out about previously taboo subjects, testing new theological waters, and urging revision of commonly accepted ideas about human sexuality is salutary. (Our protagonists, after all, laudably insist that sex can be spiritual, that desire is malleable, that sex is not the same for men and women.) For too long, theologians have construed sex, desire, and love narrowly and dogmatically, alienating and hurting many persons.

Contemporary Discourse about Sexuality

Both the feminist and Christian communities have recently made significant contributions to public discourse about sexuality in their insistence that human sexuality in many forms is a good gift, a natural and beautiful part of God's creation. The gendered nature of sexuality has also received more notice of late, with the public becoming increasingly aware of how profound the differences between men's and women's experiences of sex can be. Finally, feminist and Christian communities have both begun documenting the ways that power and violence can infuse human sexuality, resulting in the sexual abuse of children, women, and other vulnerable people. All of this work on human sexuality has had a genuinely liberating

---

3. Sharon Thompson, "Search for Tomorrow: Feminism and the Reconstruction of Teen Romance," in *Pleasure and Danger: Exploring Female Sexuality,* ed. Carole S. Vance (Boston: Routledge & Kegan Paul, 1984), 375–77.

effect, made possible by a willingness among feminists and Christians to be open to ever wider meanings and interpretations of sexual experience.

The meaning of sexuality, however, is even more complex than is currently acknowledged. The record of good work by recent Christian and feminist thinkers makes it all the more ironic to hear some of them casting their own new understandings of human sexuality in such absolute terms. No sooner do new meanings open up for what sex is *really* all about, it seems, than these become hailed as the new "true" meanings, and challenges or contradictions to them are dismissed. This interplay happens whether the truth claimed is that sexuality is a wonderful gift, a social rather than biological construct, or a political minefield.

This book focuses on a specific group of theologians — primarily Audre Lorde, Carter Heyward, Rita Nakashima Brock, Anne Bathurst Gilson, and Marvin Ellison — whose faith in a new vision of human sexuality is premature. I call them feminist theologians of the erotic. Taken together, their work represents a movement to recover the classic notion of the erotic as a drive toward fullness of life, to give this concept a feminist spin, and to proclaim that the erotic is a liberating resource which, when freed itself, will in turn remove the moral stains from human sexuality (and human life more generally). In this book I show that theologians who are attempting to put the notion of a feminist erotic to work do not finally reap as much from this notion as they claim. While their praises of the erotic have hardly destroyed sexual ethics, their overconfidence in its meaning and value is dangerous, if only because much of what they say sounds so good that one could easily overlook the weak points in their analysis. As praiseworthy as their efforts are, given the legacy these theologians are trying to dismantle, their attempt to resolve the moral problems of human sexuality by employing the erotic as a moral guide and liberatory resource does not finally succeed.

Premature faith in a vision of human sexuality becomes even more dubious when undertaking to develop a sexual ethic for adolescent girls, for the difficulty of endowing sexual experience with precise meaning becomes even more complex when considering their sexuality. Conflicting worlds of meaning for sex surround girls' moral deliberation about sexual activity. On the one hand, within many communities the assumption still operates that girls who act on their erotic impulses and desires are wrong to do so, whether because sex is dangerous terrain for them or because double standards still suggest that girls who desire sex are depraved. On the other hand, even where these assumptions are not in place, the distinction between which impulses and actions girls are free to act on and which ones are wrong has become significantly blurred. Girls still hear, for example, that they should save themselves (that is, reserve the act of intercourse) for Mr. Right, and yet they see the scorn men give to women who wait. In other words, the ethics of sexual choice are not at all clear to girls, despite how keen girls are for guidance. By and large, adolescent girls are preoccupied with doing the right thing, not only out of concern for their reputations, but also out of genuine debate over the place that intercourse will occupy in their lives.

Prior to the so-called sexual revolution of the 1960s and 1970s, the parameters for sex were more straightforward to adolescent girls. They did not generally have to discern the place of intercourse in their lives because girls were expected to marry their first lovers and start families; hence, first intercourse was assumed to go hand in hand with marriage and child rearing. Correspondingly, prior to the 1970s, most Americans shared the moral belief that marriage was the only allowable venue for sexual intercourse. Society effectively maintained this moral consensus in several ways: First, the lack of contraception controlled the incidence of teenage intercourse, and second, when girls did have sex and become pregnant, they were encouraged either to marry or to go away to a home for unwed mothers to have their babies and give them up for adoption. Adolescent marriage and homes for unwed mothers both reflected and enforced the sexual morality of their time. Both institutions ceased to flourish, however, once contraception became available to teenagers and mores began to change during the late 1960s and 1970s. Intercourse and pregnancy were themselves separated, and both were separated from marriage.[4] Therefore, when girls ask themselves today what they are reserving intercourse for, marriage is no longer the only answer and they must invent their own.

No standard has clearly replaced marriage as the *telos* of sex, so little agreement exists about the conditions under which young people should engage in sexual activity. Whether partners should wait until they are "in love," or simply mindful of each other's wishes, for example, varies from

---

4. For historical analyses of teenage pregnancy, see Rosalind Pollack Petchesky, *Abortion and Women's Choice: The State, Sexuality and Reproductive Freedom* (New York: Longman, 1984), esp. the chapter "Abortion and Heterosexual Culture: The Teenage Question"; and Laurie Schwab Zabin and Sarah C. Hayward, *Adolescent Sexual Behavior and Childbearing* (Newbury Park, Calif.: Sage Publications, 1993).

subculture to subculture. In fact, the question of when to engage in intercourse is no longer so pressing and is increasingly replaced by other moral questions. The spread of AIDS into the adolescent community during the last decade has prompted the emergence of its clearest rival consensus: Now, the decision with the most moral weight appears to be the adolescents' choice whether to have protected or unprotected sex. But even this moral distinction is not universally recognized; this consideration becomes significant primarily within liberal communities like college campuses where the permissiveness of sexual intercourse is already widespread and AIDS prevention is encouraged. In other communities, the moral difference between protected and unprotected sex is moot (or even decided in favor of *un*protected sex, as in communities where — for better or worse — the prospect of adolescent pregnancy causes less concern). In short, where once consensus about adolescent sexual activity held sway, now many competing claims upon its meaning and morality abound.[5]

Sharon Thompson's summary of the interview data for her research into adolescent sex and romance in America during the decade of the late 1970s to late 1980s helps us appreciate how girls have navigated the waters of rival sexual standards:

> Contrary to frequent pronouncements by social scientists and historians, and despite the changes of the 1970s, the double standard remained virulently alive and well, albeit less strict. According to the old double standard, when boys went all the way, they were just being boys; when girls did, they were bad. By the late 1970s, going all the way no longer definitively separated good girls from bad or boys from girls, but that didn't put an end to distinctions between those categories. Instead, distinctions multiplied. . . . [A]lthough groups of girls frequently agreed among themselves as to what constituted good and bad, there wasn't even general agreement among girls in a particular neighborhood or suburb. . . .
>
> Fashioned by girls out of the scraps and relics of previous traditions from Victorianism to sex radicalism, these fine lines in effect

---

5. These paragraphs should not be interpreted as arguing that the actual sexual behavior of adolescents has changed dramatically. That teenagers have always had sexual intercourse, and have always risked pregnancy — in not insignificant numbers — can be demonstrated by statistics. To cite just one example: Nearly one in ten girls between the ages of fifteen and nineteen gave birth in 1957. Maris A. Vinovskis, "An 'Epidemic' of Adolescent Pregnancy? Some Historical Considerations," *Journal of Family History* 6, no. 2 (summer 1981): 208. I am arguing that the moral meaning assigned to adolescent sexual behavior has changed.

constituted local and individual sex and gender subsystems. They gave girls maps on which to orient themselves (no small matter in a culture that advertises sexuality as comprising the essence of self) and rationalized sexual losses: As a result girls found these constructions extremely helpful, and perpetuated and multiplied them.[6]

Adolescent girls still struggle today to construct moral meaning for their sexual experiences. Their earnest desire for a moral map in a disorienting world should not lead feminist theologians and ethicists to present sexuality in any overly simplified way. In particular, the persistent effects of gender inequality upon sexual experience should not be minimized but rather examined in fresh ways. Female adolescent sexuality simply cannot be understood apart from the dynamics of gender, power, and culture, which are not easily teased apart.

Considerations for a Sexual Ethic for Adolescence

In developing a sexual ethic for adolescence, feminist theologians and ethicists should keep at least three considerations in mind. Let me present these considerations as corrections to feminist theologies of the erotic. One correction would be to replace the kind of absolutism and confidence found in these theologies with genuine and open inquiry into the diversity of meanings that young people ascribe to sexuality. Feminist theologians of the erotic base their vision of the erotic on a limited range of human experiences, especially those of adult women who to a great degree have already been "liberated." To correct this tendency, we need to listen to a wide plurality of voices, inviting multiple thick descriptions of the actual varied desires, joys, and tragedies of female sexual experience. In part, we simply need more of the kind of data Sharon Thompson has collected about what patterns exist in girls' actual experience. If girls tell us that the meaning of sexuality is still far from settled in their lives, then we know that the revolution feminist theologians of the erotic have been attempting to bring about has not yet fully succeeded.

Girls' testimony also warns us not simply to replace older, inadequate ideologies with newer, "better" ones and even to avoid ideology altogether. This caveat may be especially true regarding ideologies about "the

---

6. Sharon Thompson, *Going All the Way: Teenage Girls' Tales of Sex, Romance, and Pregnancy* (New York: Hill and Wang, 1995), 31–32.

erotic." If feminist theologies of the erotic have already successfully rendered theological discourse about the erotic more positive and inclusive — so that the erotic is no longer viewed merely as an embarrassing eruption but as an overtly passionate drive suffusing many aspects of human life — then the next step should be to acknowledge that its content might never be completely stable or fixed but always produced by social conditions (such as gendered double standards). A second correction, in other words, would be a decentering of our own assumptions about what adolescents find erotic and why. We need to theorize about the complexities and ironies of erotic life, to make sense of the erotic's many faces and sometimes its absence. We must admit that however much we want to affirm the goodness of the erotic, it may not always be entirely seemly and may occasionally be maddening. While denigrating the erotic as a mere animalistic urge may now be foolish, swinging in the other direction and glorifying the erotic as always kind is equally unwise. While it may no longer be taboo, neither will the erotic ever be the key to all liberation.

Decentering the meaning of human sexuality does not mean that sexual ethics cannot offer critique of certain choices and work toward the transformation of sexual relationships that are harmful and debilitating. Actually sexual ethics must perform exactly this function. The rationale for doing any kind of ethics, after all, is the conviction that better and worse ways to construct human life do exist; identifying them is the ethicists' work. But too much of the current work in sexual ethics, especially the work I am calling feminist theology of the erotic, remains content to set forth new visions, or "articles of transcendent faith," as Sands puts it. Unfortunately, even the most ardently voiced convictions about what Eros is really all about are ultimately unsatisfying. Conviction without theory is inadequate.[7] In addition to expressing convictions about how young people *ought* to conduct their sexual lives, ethics needs to incorporate theories about why the erotic assumes particular contours in young people's lives. How should their descriptions of experience be interpreted? How is the erotic produced and reproduced in such similar ways over and over again in adolescent girls' lives? How do some erotic yearnings get "under the skin" and lodge there? Why do girls perceive their choices to be so limited? What prevents many girls and women from realizing the liberat-

---

7. "A conviction is not a theory, however," reminds Mary McClintock Fulkerson in *Changing the Subject: Women's Discourses and Feminist Theology* (Minneapolis: Fortress Press, 1994), 42.

ing feminist vision that seems obvious to others? Without addressing such theoretical questions, any moral advice to adolescent girls about sexual relationship remains idealistic and insubstantial. Feminist theologies of the erotic tend to rest on outdated theories about women's experience, even women's erotic experience. We need to replace these theories.

A third correction would be to supply moral norms that befit the reality of proliferating standards for sexual experience. Feminist theologies of the erotic offer insufficient normative content, relying as they do on visionary statements to inspire and motivate women and men. We need to offer something different. A pragmatic sexual ethic would be fitting. We can and should help clarify for young people the relational patterns that tend to enable flourishing and those that tend to disable and constrain. Given that worlds of meaning will continue to shift while adolescents continue to have sex, a better approach may be to cast their sexual relationships as occasions for vulnerability that are nevertheless also occasions for pleasure.

Acknowledging that sexual life is a morally ambiguous mixture of pleasure and pain does not concede too much. Most people, after all, find that no singular meaning or purpose for sexuality endures over the course of their entire life. They find that the texture and shape of sexual experience are too rich and varied. Experientially, what thrills a person erotically at one time often leaves them bored later. Pleasure and pain are often curiously mixed, even sometimes indistinguishable. Furthermore, the nature and purpose of sexuality are difficult to pinpoint philosophically. The two persistent themes of sexual experience may simply be its intensity and the attending risk of vulnerability. (These truths may be the only two we can affirm with certainty.) In sexual experience we encounter, as Ricoeur says, all the human difficulties, gropings, dangers, dilemmas, failures, and joys. Thus, sweeping claims about the moral meaning of sexuality can no longer be justified and more limited claims might serve as worthy replacements. Given the multiplicity and unpredictability of human sexual experience, what people need most by way of normative content is a way to reduce the risk of needless vulnerability in their sexual relationship. For adolescents who are just encountering the world of sexual experience, practical guidance for minimizing risk is especially important.

Although feminist theologies of the erotic have only inadequately pursued these three corrections (creating multiple, thick descriptions of erotic experience; updating the theoretical assumptions that have heretofore undergirded sexual ethics; and eschewing grand moral claims in favor of practical moral guidance), certain other feminist theologians whose work inspires the present study have indeed undertaken to discover needed changes. Rebecca Chopp is one example. As she outlines it, the journey of feminist theology in our time requires at least three moves, which correspond to the corrections just presented: First, reading the actual situations of many women for thick descriptions of life lived under the oppression of patriarchy; second, analyzing the productive and reproductive relationships between individual experience and social institutions; and third, moving beyond ideological critique toward discourses of radical transformation.[8]

Constructing a Sexual Ethic for Adolescent Girls

In this book I cannot, of course, accomplish everything outlined; within limits, I engage in all three corrections, after first summarizing, critiquing, and historically situating feminist theologies of the erotic. To thicken the description of female adolescent erotic experience, I examine empirical evidence from the lives of teenage girls. Listening carefully to their stories, I draw a comparison between what they say — and do not say — about the erotic with what feminist theologians have proclaimed. This comparison reveals that feminist theologians are altogether too confident about the possibilities for erotic liberation — not so much because girls are unfamiliar with the power of the erotic, but because they are constrained *as girls* by the power of gender. To add theoretical depth to my interpretation of girls' erotic experience, I draw upon feminist psychological and psychoanalytic theories. These theories provide not only a helpful way to read the empirical evidence but also an explanation of how the erotic is constructed for girls and women. In other words, the theories underscore why any claims about the erotic must reckon seriously with the perpetual effects of gender on Eros. Finally, to begin formulating helpful norms for sexual relationship, I propose a discourse of vulnerability and trust rather than one of Eros and liberation. The erotic alone will not liberate girls and women; rather, relations of power need to be transformed so

8. Rebecca Chopp, "Seeing and Naming the World Anew: The Works of Rosemary Radford Ruether," *Religious Studies Review* 15, no. 1 (January 1989): 1–11. See also Chopp's "Feminism's Theological Pragmatics: A Social Naturalism of Women's Experience," *Journal of Religion* 67, no. 2 (April 1987): 239–56. There, she proposes a "feminist pragmatics of inquiry" that would include a situated, rather than essential, view of knowledge; an "exploration into the full complexity of reality"; and a commitment to transforming oppressive social conditions.

that females are liberated into a just rather than an unjust order.[9] In the meantime, sexual partners need to acknowledge the interpersonal vulnerability that comes with Eros and try to develop erotic relationships that appropriately embody trust.

At this point, a brief outline of the content of each chapter and its contribution to the overall project can help the reader. Chapter 2 introduces the movement in sexual theology and ethics that I am calling feminist theologies of the erotic. The chapter first identifies common themes and arguments in these theologies, then examines selected works of five representative theologians.

Chapter 3 develops a critique of feminist theologies of the erotic by placing them alongside two different sets of conversation partners: first, contemporary secular theorists whose discourse about sexuality is much less sanguine; and second, even earlier theologians within the field of feminist theology. The latter comparison shows that the primary reason feminist theologians of the erotic sound so confident is that they are deliberately challenging older, liberal feminist assumptions about the similarity between men's and women's experience and promoting instead the idea that women's experience is uniquely revelatory.

Chapter 4 examines accounts of the erotic offered by teenage girls who were the subjects of a psychologist, a social historian, and journalists for studies on adolescent sexuality. These interviews contain two challenges to feminist theologies of the erotic. On the one hand, many adolescent girls become perplexed and anxious when asked about their erotic experience, despite their familiarity with feminism and their willingness to report their sexual activity. In effect, girls tell interviewers that expressing eroticism contradicts what dominant culture still teaches them about being female (in a way that merely having sex does not). Cultural expectations lead them to silence their desires either for or against sex, and to defer instead to their male partners' desires. To make erotic choices is to transgress a gender role. Even to contemplate such transgression produces perplexity and anxiety. On the other hand, many girls also report that romance lures them, and they avidly choose romantic entanglements. They recognize this desire, too, as a gendered one. Despite their knowledge that it rarely

9. This book does not develop a theory of sexuality and justice because Margaret Farley is already doing that. She was the first within the feminist theological community to articulate a need for a theory of justice in sexual ethics. See her *Just Love: Sexual Ethics and Social Change* (New York: Crossroad, 1998).

brings fullness of life, girls yearn for romantic involvement. Romance effectively becomes the meaning of "the erotic" for some of them.

Chapter 5 examines the construction of female adolescent Eros. The discussion focuses on the thesis that girls' experiences of anxiety and ambivalence, as well as their intense interest in romantic relationship, are linked to issues in the development of the female self. Learning to be female, at least within the gender-structured families that dominate contemporary U.S. society, conflicts with learning to be differentiated, independent, and self-confident — and yet healthy self-development requires both. Therefore, girls unconsciously employ various strategies to resolve the conflict. The strategies they employ, it turns out, account for the anxious silence and self-disavowal that often characterize their discourse about the erotic. Girls' struggle to become separate selves also explains their preoccupation with relational issues. Chapter 5 reports, in other words, on good reasons that girls and women cannot and should not simply place more faith in their erotic experience, as feminist theologians of the erotic would have them do.

Chapter 6 turns to the question of what kind of sexual ethic befits the more chastened, sober view of Eros presented in this book. The chapter suggests that sexual relationships be viewed from the perspective of interpersonal trust and examines both an ethos of trust and an ethos of distrust relative to this kind of relationship. If, as I argue, the moral problems associated with sexuality are less sex-negativity and repression of the erotic than ambiguity within the meaning of the erotic, then the appropriate norm for sexual practices is one that will not so much liberate as protect sexual partners. Whether the norm is guarded trust or healthy distrust depends on the level of vulnerability within the relationship. Practical guidance about appropriate levels of trust is preferable to the imprecise idealism of feminist theologies of the erotic. Chapter 7 evaluates the conclusions of this project and points toward future lines of inquiry regarding this topic.

While others who are working to reformulate Christian sexual ethics and feminist theological ethics are my primary conversation partners in this project, I indirectly incorporate other conversations as well. I share the concerns of people in other disciplines who debate the nature of human sexuality in general and female sexuality in particular. Religious feminists have remained remarkably detached from the "sex wars" that divide secular feminist theorists into "pro-sex" and "radical" camps, or "pleasure"

and "danger" theories, respectively.[10] Granted, these debates have sometimes created more heat than light; nevertheless, detachment from them
unfortunately means that Christian feminists writing on sexuality are not
full partners in dialogue with the rest of the feminist community.

Another marriage that has generally failed to flourish is that between
theological ethicists and psychoanalytic theorists. Because psychoanalytic
theory makes a potentially significant contribution to theories of moral
motivation, this disconnect is regrettable.[11] But a cursory glance at the
publications in which object relations theory, for example, is currently
being applied to religious studies suggests that it remains mainly of interest to pastoral theologians and phenomenologists of religion. This book
makes one small contribution to furthering the use of psychoanalytic
theory in the field of ethics.[12]

My recommendation in this book that Christian feminists not uncritically valorize female relationality positions me alongside moral theorists
who resist the characterization of women as more caring and relational. At
the same time, my argument that many adolescent girls *do* become more
preoccupied with relationship reveals my sympathy for theories about the
commonality of female experience. Thus, the argument embraces postmodernist reservations about essentialism as well as modernist insistence
that difference needs to be explained. This debate is related also to debates in moral theory about care versus justice and the situated versus
autonomous self, so those issues resonate in the background of this book
as well.[13]

Skepticism and postmodernism have touched philosophical and theo-

---

10. Sands, "Uses of the Thea(o)logian," 9.

11. Ernest Wallwork criticizes the lukewarm interest contemporary ethicists display in a moral
psychology that takes psychology and psychoanalysis seriously. "[S]o far, this renewed interest
has failed to bring forth any serious engagement by ethicists with psychoanalysis...." Ernest
Wallwork, *Psychoanalysis and Ethics* (New Haven: Yale University Press, 1991), 7.

12. Diana Jonte-Pace suggests that scholars of religious studies might take interest in some of
the recent texts on psychoanalysis and feminism. "Regardless of the absence of explicit attention
to religion in these texts, there is rich material here for scholars of religion.... [Jessica] Benjamin's analysis of the desire for recognition in the origins of the structures of domination and
submission points toward a new encounter between feminist psychoanalysis and ethics." Diana
Jonte-Pace, "Psychoanalysis after Feminism," *Religious Studies Review* 19, no. 2 (April 1993): 114.

13. See Seyla Benhabib, *Situating the Self: Gender, Community, and Postmodernism in Con-
temporary Ethics* (New York: Routledge, 1992), especially the essays, "The Generalized and the
Concrete Other: The Kohlberg-Gilligan Controversy and Moral Theory" and "The Debate over
Women and Moral Theory Revisited." See also Diana Meyers, "The Socialized Individual and In-
dividual Autonomy: An Intersection between Philosophy and Psychology," in *Women and Moral
Theory,* ed. Eva Feder Kittay and Diana T. Meyers (Totowa, N.J.: Rowman and Littlefield, 1987).

logical ethics in many ways. My emphasis in this book on sexuality's multiple meanings indicates acceptance of diverse and even fragmented centers of value in the moral life more generally. My preference for an ethic of trust rather than some kind of rule-based sexual morality recognizes that a single moral theory is difficult to justify anymore but that persons still need normative guidance for sexual conduct.[14]

The attempt to weave several discourses together characterizes much contemporary feminist ethics, and this book is no exception. My aim is to achieve some degree of wisdom and insight that might ultimately help young people, girls in particular, through the difficulties, dangers, and dilemmas of their lives.

---

14. Among many possible references, significant ones include Thomas Nagel, "The Fragmentation of Value," in *Mortal Questions* (Cambridge: Cambridge University Press, 1979); and Annette C. Baier, *Moral Prejudices: Essays on Ethics* (Cambridge, Mass.: Harvard University Press, 1994).

TWO

Regarding the Erotic
as Solution

If love is the answer, could you please rephrase the question?
— Lily Tomlin

SPEAKING AT MOUNT HOLYOKE COLLEGE in 1978 at a conference
on the history of women, Audre Lorde confidently proclaimed that
the erotic could transform lives. For Lorde, the erotic was the most important source of joy, power, and creative energy in women's lives — "the
knowledge and use of which we are now reclaiming in our language,
our history, our dancing, our loving, our work, our lives."[1] She called
upon women to "reassess the very quality of [their] lives" in all aspects,
including sensual, spiritual, and political. Lorde spoke eloquently of her
own discovery of the joys that had opened to her once she awakened to
the erotic: The erotic "fearless[ly] underlined [her] capacity for joy." She
claimed to feel the erotic in potentially every activity: "In the way my
body stretches to music and opens into response, hearkening to its deepest rhythms, so every level upon which I sense also opens to the erotically
satisfying experience, whether it is dancing, building a bookcase, writing
a poem, examining an idea."[2] She predicted that the erotic could connect
private pleasure to political action:

> For as we begin to recognize our deepest feelings, we begin to give
> up, of necessity, being satisfied with suffering and self-abnegation,
> and with the numbness which so often seems like their only alterna-
> tive in our society. Our acts against oppression become integral with
> self, motivated and empowered from within.[3]

1. Audre Lorde, "Uses of the Erotic: The Erotic as Power," in *Sister Outsider: Essays and
Speeches by Audre Lorde* (Trumansburg, N.Y.: Crossing Press, 1984), 53–59.
2. Lorde, "Uses of the Erotic," 56–57.
3. Lorde, "Uses of the Erotic," 58.

16

Lorde's speech was later published as a pamphlet that gained widespread popular attention in activist circles. Her comments also struck a chord within academic feminism, both religious and secular. A movement to recover Eros, or "the erotic," began to gather steam in feminist theology and feminist theological ethics, claiming the importance of Eros and calling for its liberation from captivity in human life.[4] As previously noted, I call this work feminist theology of the erotic.[5] Feminist theologians and ethicists have developed a set of themes about the erotic that has become a common refrain: The erotic is a fundamental drive toward fullness of life that all persons possess but which has for too long been misunderstood and maligned. This negative legacy needs to be overturned. Fearing the erotic is not necessary because it is inherently good; only its distortions are bad. The (genuine) erotic should be nurtured, celebrated, and even exploited, for it has the power to enhance rather than diminish human flourishing. Indeed, in touch with the erotic within, women and men can overcome oppressions such as sexism and sexual repression that prevent their full flourishing as human beings. Therefore, the power of the erotic should function as an internal resource for sexual, psychic, spiritual, and political transformation. To liberate the erotic is to liberate the person.

Anyone working in the area of theological sexual ethics must reckon with this proliferating discourse about the erotic. Has the turn in this direction been entirely positive for sexual ethics? I argue that it has not —

---

4. Different writers use the terms "Eros" and "the erotic." For my purposes here, the terms are interchangeable.

5. In addition to Lorde, see J. Michael Clark, *A Defiant Celebration: Theological Ethics and Gay Sexuality* (Garland, Tex.: Tangelwuld, 1990); Paula Cooey, Sharon Farmer, and Mary Ellen Ross, eds., *Embodied Love: Sensuality and Relationship as Feminist Values* (San Francisco: Harper & Row, 1988); Marvin Ellison, *Erotic Justice: A Liberating Ethic of Sexuality* (Louisville, Ky.: Westminster/John Knox Press, 1996); Carter Heyward, *The Redemption of God: A Theology of Mutual Relation* (Lanham, Md.: University Press of America, 1982), *Our Passion for Justice: Images of Power, Sexuality, and Liberation* (New York: Pilgrim Press, 1984), and *Touching Our Strength: The Erotic as Power and the Love of God* (San Francisco: HarperSanFrancisco, 1989); Rita Nakashima Brock, *Journeys by Heart: A Christology of Erotic Power* (New York: Crossroad, 1988); James Nelson, *Embodiment: An Approach to Sexuality and Christian Theology* (Minneapolis: Augsburg Publishing House, 1978), *Between Two Gardens: Reflections on Sexuality and Religious Experience* (Cleveland: Pilgrim Press, 1983), *The Intimate Connection: Male Sexuality, Masculine Spirituality* (Philadelphia: Westminster Press, 1988), and *Body Theology* (Louisville, Ky.: Westminster/John Knox Press, 1992), Part One; James Nelson and Sandra Longfellow, eds., *Sexuality and the Sacred: Sources for Theological Reflection* (Louisville, Ky.: Westminster/John Knox Press, 1994); Judith Plaskow, *Standing Again at Sinai: Judaism from a Feminist Perspective* (San Francisco: Harper Collins, 1990), chap. 5; Anne Bathurst Gilson, *Eros Breaking Free: Interpreting Sexual Theo-Ethics* (Cleveland: Pilgrim Press, 1995).

that, in fact, the time has come to move beyond theologies of the erotic toward a more pragmatic ethics of sexual relationship.

Meanings of the Erotic

Gaining an overview of feminist theological discourse about the erotic can be useful because it will enhance understanding of "the erotic" as well as the claims being made for how the erotic should ideally function in human life. When attempting to identify and summarize a discourse, one runs the risk of unjustified generalization. I therefore endeavor to point out subtleties and differences among writers whenever possible. Nonetheless, a fair statement is that most feminist theologies of the erotic mean one or more of the following when they refer to the erotic: Love, sensuality, wisdom, or relationality.[6] When feminist theologies name the erotic as love, they are emphasizing the closeness and intimacy of erotic relationships. As sensuality, they are naming women's and men's power to reach greater depths of passion and joy. Naming the erotic as wisdom suggests that it awakens greater understanding of oppression and possibilities for liberation. As relationality, the erotic is said to tighten the bonds of mutuality between people. These four ways of naming what is "erotic" about human life have become four hallmarks of feminist theological discourse about the erotic.

Such discourse assumes the erotic to be a powerful, innate drive that has the potential to set human persons free. One way of interpreting the discourse is as a revival of ancient understandings of the erotic.[7] For Plato, Eros was a drive toward fullness of life. In the *Symposium,* we hear Aristophanes defining Eros as the search for one's missing half; hence the ageless theme of love as union — or even *re*-union — goes back to Plato. Socrates adds the qualification that the goodness of the other is the true object of the search. Putting the two together, we get Plato's classic

---

6. Alexander Irwin's analysis of many of the same theologians has influenced me here. He reads feminist and womanist theologies as making five basic claims about Eros: Eros is joy; Eros is a source of knowledge; Eros is relational; Eros is a cosmic force; and Eros is political. See Alexander C. Irwin, "Eros and 'Power in Right Relation': The Erotic in Feminist and Womanist Theologies," *Eros toward the World: Paul Tillich and the Theology of the Erotic* (Minneapolis: Fortress Press, 1991).

7. See John Burnaby, "Love: Historical Perspectives," in *The Westminster Dictionary of Christian Ethics,* ed. James F. Childress and John Macquarrie (Philadelphia: Westminster Press, 1986), and Gene Outka, "Love" in the *Encyclopedia of Ethics,* ed. Lawrence C. Becker and Charlotte Becker (New York: Garland Publications Inc., 1992), 742–51.

formula that love is desire for the perpetual possession of the good. Plato also treats the theme of love in the *Phaedrus,* where, using the metaphor of a charioteer's two horses straining in different directions, he highlights the tension between the soul's aspiration for true goodness or beauty versus the soul's desire for earthly, material objects.[8]

Feminist theologians of the erotic, however, unlike Plato, insist that the erotic always has liberatory potential, that negative forces only temporarily hold the erotic captive. We see later that contemporary feminist theological discourse about the erotic both retrieves and corrects important features of philosophical and theological discourse about Eros. The correcting impulse tends to overshadow the retrieving with ambiguous results. In the order I have introduced them, the four ways of naming the erotic (love, sensuality, wisdom, and relationality) represent increasing departures from traditional views of Eros because of progressively novel claims about the functioning and power of the erotic. At the same time, the latter descriptions of the erotic also become more problematic for feminists because they reinforce constructions of femininity that now frequently come under question. While feminist theologians of the erotic are correct to insist that distortions of the meaning of the erotic contribute to problems in human sexuality (and other arenas of human life as well), they go too far in maintaining the notion that a liberated "erotic" can solve all the problems they claim.

The Erotic as Love

When feminist theologians of the erotic call the erotic "love," they remain more or less faithful to traditional discourses. That is to say, in this guise the feminist "erotic" bears a basic resemblance to the *Eros* of Western philosophy and theology. "Eros" is the name traditionally given to the kind of love or passion that is elicited by, and moves people toward, the objects they desire. Used in its original sense, the term "Eros" refers to an acquisitive love — a love whose aim is, in one way or another, possession.[9] Eros is characterized as a force or drive, one that propels people to satisfy deep and intense desires, to seek after and possess whatever they perceive will lead to their fulfillment. While every kind of love seeks satisfaction,

---

8. For a full discussion of Plato's doctrine of Eros, see Irving Singer, *The Nature of Love,* vol. 1 (Chicago: University of Chicago Press, 1984).

9. Outka writes that Eros is "desire for the good, fulfilled when one possesses the good in perpetuity." Outka, "Love," 742.

the term "Eros" has been reserved for love that has an insistent, driving quality and the explicit goal of self-satisfaction. Other forms of love, especially Philia and Agape, focus more on the *other's* satisfaction. As Gene Outka puts it, as we move away from purely erotic love, "the accent falls away on one's own possession."[10] Perceived as a "drive" because of its animating force, Eros is summoned by the beauty of particular objects and stirs the human person to reach outward in response. Eros is active, moving people toward unity and connection and likened to an impulse or energizing source.

The object of Eros's desire is frequently assumed to be another person. Therefore Eros is linked to personal attraction. But Eros transcends mere lust. Unlike Epithymia, traditionally understood as the libidinal human desire for pleasure satisfaction, Eros drives the lover toward satisfaction by beauty or good itself. Eros has always signified more than mere arousal or the desire to experience sexual pleasure with another person, signifying instead a fundamental and essential human yearning for union. Insofar as all persons feel somehow incomplete without possessing the beauty and goodness of other human beings, this longing for completion could bear the name Eros. Sometimes in the tradition, Eros is also described as love for nonhuman objects. Some thinkers claim the possibility of loving erotically other creatures, inanimate objects, institutions, activities, and even ideas. They so argue because, again, if Eros is simply the drive toward fullness of life, presumably whatever is life-fulfilling can be desired erotically.

Feminist theologians of the erotic share this understanding of Eros. For them, Eros/the erotic is that enlivening energy that puts an individual in touch with self, others, and world. So, for example, Carter Heyward describes the erotic as "the basis of our capacity to participate in mutually empowering relationships."[11] Feminists share the traditional definition of the erotic as a passion that transcends mere physical desire. In fact, they often define " the erotic" *very* widely, using the term to talk about passions for justice, community, and so on. We have already glimpsed the wide scope of "erotic love" in Lorde's speech. The erotic, she said, awakened her to a multitude of joys and passions simultaneously sensual, interpersonal, and spiritual. Heyward, one of the primary feminist theologians to

---

10. Outka, "Love," 742.
11. Heyward, *Touching Our Strength,* 187.

champion the recovery of the erotic, insists that the erotic encompasses love for whatever makes one more alive. She uses the language of the erotic for everything from physical feelings and sensations, deep affection for a beloved and longings for intimacy to capacities for self-awareness:

> The erotic is our desire to taste and smell and see and hear and touch one another. It's our yearning to be involved — all "rolled up" — in each other's sounds and glances and bodies and feelings. The erotic is the flow of our senses, in which we experience our bodies' power and desire to connect with others. The erotic moves transpersonally among us and also draws us more fully into ourselves.[12]

Feminist theologians of the erotic typically conflate many different meanings this way. Judith Plaskow says that the erotic feeling which binds members of a community is at once intellectual and sexual. "True intellectual exchange, common work, shared experience are laced with sexual energy that animates and enlivens them," she writes, explaining why love for the community is erotic love.[13] Rita Nakashima Brock, on the other hand, takes pains to distance her definition of erotic love from sexuality. In Brock's work on the erotic and its relationship to Christology, she retrieves and revives the part of the tradition that emphasizes the universal connection-building function of Eros. The erotic for her becomes that psychological drive toward relationship or connection with others. In fact, she defines the erotic as connection. "Erotic power is the fundamental power of existence-as-a-relational-process."[14]

Traditional discourse about erotic love has always been somewhat ambivalent about love that is too passionate, too driven. Western thinkers have tended to voice faintly their praise for Eros. They mute or qualify their affirmation of a love with too many erotic connotations. Any passion that carries power and intensity philosophers and theologians have regarded with some suspicion. The supposed insatiability of Eros has won it the reputation of being a dangerous form of love. In the Christian tradition, which has created a typology of loves, Eros has historically emerged lower in value than Agape and Philia, Agape being neighbor-love that is

---

12. Heyward, *Touching Our Strength*, 187.
13. Plaskow, *Standing Again at Sinai*, 201.
14. Brock, *Journeys by Heart*, 41. Brock also moves beyond tradition by identifying the erotic with the figure of Christ/Christa.

unilateral, unconditional, unmotivated, and universal in scope, and Philia being friendship-love that is fond, caring, and well-wishing.

Theologians have traditionally denigrated Eros because love that is overly acquisitive arouses their suspicion. Such a love runs the risk of overwhelming the lover and the beloved while also reinforcing lovers' natural inclination to satisfy themselves rather than others. Augustine says that only love for God is ultimately satisfying, as his famous utterances in the Confessions demonstrate: "Our hearts find no peace until they rest in you" and "Love is the weight by which I act." In City of God, he promotes Caritas as the love that directs us upward toward God rather than downward into sin, as in the passage, "In Him our existence will know no death, our knowledge embrace no error, our love meet no resistance." Aquinas says that all human loves should be referred finally to God.[15] Christian theologians worry that love should bestow rather than acquire value. Many people would interpret Jesus' question to his followers in this fashion: "[I]f you love those who love you, what reward have you?"[16] They worry that Eros might not do anything but mire a person in trivial and selfish desires and wonder whether a passion so consuming can be moral. For Plato, the driving nature of Eros could only be justified by harnessing its power to the soul's aspiration for the highest good; ever since Plato, philosophers and theologians have attempted to reconcile Eros's seeming selfishness and irrepressibility with love's goal of reaching beyond itself. In the Christian tradition, such concerns could be said to have reached their zenith in the work of Lutheran theologian Anders Nygren, whose contempt for the inclusion of Eros in the typology of Christian loves was profound. For Nygren, Agape and Eros are not merely distinct forms of love, but "dangerous rivals."[17]

Recently, however, many theologians have come to regard exaggerated suspicions of Eros as outdated and overblown. Eros is increasingly accorded higher status in Christian ethical discourse. Frequent calls are made for a balance among the different types of love and even some assertions of equality. For example, several Christian theologians and ethicists have attempted in recent years to demonstrate that Eros is compatible with

---

15. Augustine's *Confessions* (1.1) and (13.9), respectively; Augustine, *City of God* (11.28); Thomas Aquinas, *Summa Theologica* II-II, q. 24.

16. Matthew 5:46, Revised Standard Version.

17. Anders Nygren, *Agape and Eros*, trans. Philip Watson (Philadelphia: Westminster Press, 1953), 162.

Agape; some people have even ventured to say that the former is essential to Christian neighbor-love.[18] The writers whom I am calling feminist theologians of the erotic applaud the direction theological discourse is taking in this regard. They, too, attempt to resolve theology's historic ambivalence about erotic love. As one might expect, these authors constitute some of the most vigorous proponents today of the positive value of erotic love in human life.

When naming the erotic as love, feminist theologians of the erotic borrow many of the tradition's historic meanings of Eros but do not share the tradition's skepticism. If Western philosophers and theologians have traditionally muted their praise of erotic love, feminist theologians of the erotic trumpet theirs. The erotic, for them, is not the problem but the solution. They argue that satisfying one's own yearnings for beauty and goodness does not detract from one's moral and spiritual life. On the contrary, they insist that erotic passions nurture the self and therefore also, indirectly, others. They do not see the erotic as selfish; rather, Eros represents for them the basic human yearning to flourish and find completion and happiness; they insist that women and men should encourage the "release" of the erotic. They reject the idea that erotic love demeans the lover or harms the beloved, and in fact claim just the opposite: To love erotically does not contradict, and may even fulfill, agapeic love. Heyward goes so far as to argue that the erotic is the epitome of Christian love of God: "The erotic is our most fully embodied experience of the love of God.... Regardless of who may be the lovers, the root of the love is sacred movement between and among us."[19]

Some theologians of the erotic argue that the supposed contradiction between erotic love and "higher" forms of love is not only misleading but also prevents people from seeing that the erotic supplies unique ethical norms. While Agape stresses fairness and impartiality, Eros stresses mutuality and connection. If people only loved agapeically, they would miss this dimension, also integral to the moral life.

In summary, feminist theologies of the erotic seek to claim for Eros the positive reputation that has traditionally been reserved for other forms of love and seek to align the erotic with the ethical and the spiritual. Drawing

---

18. See the discussion among Colin Grant, "For the Love of God"; Carter Heyward, "Lamenting the Loss of Love"; and Edward Vacek, "Love: Christian and Diverse," in the *Journal of Religious Ethics* 24, no. 1 (spring 1996).

19. Heyward, *Touching Our Strength*, 99.

on the classic understanding of Eros as the basic human drive toward fullness of life, they propose that the erotic is the solution to emptiness of life. Experiences of erotic love can create meaning out of meaninglessness and connection out of separation. Feminist theologians of the erotic are convinced not only that erotic love has been maligned and misunderstood but that it provides the key to overcoming human misery.

The Erotic as Sensuality

In Western traditions, Eros has usually been associated with the body and embodied passion. The erotic has a long association with sensual appetites in general and sexual appetite in particular. In ancient Greek culture, Eros was the god of sexual desire, symbolizing a mysterious and irresistible power that overtakes and controls lovers. While Eros eventually took on meaning wider than physical passion (as stated above), at least some reference to the body has invariably remained. Passion awakened by and expressed through the senses of touch, sight, hearing, smell, and taste is called "erotic." Erotic love is often assumed to mature through physical intimacy and to culminate in the physical (not only metaphorical) union of two individuals.

At the same time, the embodied power of Eros has instilled fear. While expressing ambivalence about the acquisitive and self-seeking side of Eros, the tradition has expressed even more about its sensuality. Strains of dualism within the Western tradition have contributed to the persistent devaluation of whatever is associated with the body, and human sensuality and sexuality have been prime targets. Embodied desires, emotions, and passions have been treated with suspicion, especially when compared to the supposedly higher faculty of human reason. Sexual desires in particular have been portrayed as uncontrollable and unpredictable, leading human persons into sin. Hence, anything associated with the erotic has been devalued as well.

Feminist theologians of the erotic lament the fear and suspicion that the body evokes. They try to recover what they take to be the original, more positive, meaning of the erotic — the sense of Eros as a warm and lively passion. In fact, feminists often praise sensual experiences in glowing terms. For example, Lorde claimed that awakening to her sensuality made her more capable of experiencing joy. She and other feminists believe, therefore, that to recover the full positive power of the erotic in their lives, men and women need even more sensual pleasure and fulfillment.

They argue that fullness of life includes, and even demands, greater access to one's own sensuality. "[The erotic] is an internal sense of satisfaction to which, once we have experienced it, we know we can aspire. For having experienced the fullness of this depth of feeling and recognizing its power, in honor and self-respect we can require no less of ourselves."[20]

In large measure, feminist theologians of the erotic part ways with traditional views of Eros precisely over the meaning ascribed to human desire. These feminist theologians object to the portrayal of desire in general and sensual desire in particular as irrepressible and uncontrollable. They also take strong exception to the equation of sensuality with sin. Feminists argue that these traditional assessments of erotic desire trace back to faulty anthropologies which see the mind or soul of the human person continuously under assault by the dangerous and irresistible impulses of the body. One can only assume that Eros is dangerous, they argue, if one assumes sensual desires to be wild impulses that always lead a person astray. A feminist anthropology of the human person, in contrast, sees mind, soul, and body in harmony with each other, not assuming that the body drags the rest of the person down or that bodily feelings themselves necessarily lead one astray. Embodied passions, according to this feminist view, no more need to be feared than other kinds of passions.

The anthropology upon which a fearful view of sensuality is based is increasingly considered inaccurate and in need of replacement by a more affirmative view of the human person as an integration of body, mind, and spirit. Yet the effects of the old anthropology linger in discourses about the erotic, and feminist theologians of the erotic labor to expose and correct them. In addition to shifting the discourse in a more positive direction, then, they direct a great deal of their energy at dismantling outdated models of the human person and human desire and demonstrating the ways in which harmful ideologies of the body continue to operate in theology and ethics.

Judith Plaskow's work affords one example. She argues that unwarranted fear, shame, and suspicion of the erotic continue to linger in Jewish theological discourse. Plaskow has a nuanced view of the erotic; she talks about it as having potential for both good and evil. She is mindful that Judaism has not warned of the danger of erotic passions for no reason. Erotic feelings, she says, especially when allowed to go unchecked, do have

---

20. Lorde, "Uses of the Erotic," 54.

the power to mislead. Nevertheless, she sounds a theme common to many other feminist theologians of the erotic: The erotic is an essential part of human nature and should therefore be wholeheartedly accepted.[21] To feel passionately — to be enlivened with erotic energy — is a positive event for a person and should be honored rather than repressed. Contrasting her own affirmation of the erotic with its suppression in patriarchal Jewish culture, she writes: "From a feminist perspective, however, the power and danger of the erotic are not reasons to fear and suppress it but to nurture it as a profound personal and communal resource in the struggle for change."[22]

More particularly, feminist theologians see a large part of their theological task to be restoring human sexuality to a place of respect and celebration. One of their most consistent critiques takes to task what they perceive to be the equation of sexual morality with sexual restraint — what they and others frequently call, in shorthand, "sex-negativity." Sex-negativity, in this sense, is the attitude or assumption that sexual passion must be restrained to be moral. This attitude toward sexuality is negative because it assumes from the start that sexual feelings are primarily bad or at least dangerous and must therefore be repressed or restrained. But repression and restraint, argue feminist theologians of the erotic, can only be morally preferable if laxity and excess are assumed to be otherwise inevitable — a view of sexual desire they reject as inaccurate. Few women, feminist theologians of the erotic point out, suffer from unrestrained sexual desire. Most women could restrain themselves less without undermining their sexual morality. Many if not most of the problems associated with sexual behavior (susceptibility to seduction and rape, for example) feminist theologians of the erotic attribute to a poverty of genuine sexual passion, not to an excess.

Feminist theologians of the erotic can make this claim because they retain the vision of sexuality as powerful and even consuming (as Plaskow's quotation above demonstrates), but claim that therein lies its strength, rather than its weakness, as has traditionally been assumed. They criticize Western tradition for confusing sexuality's power with evil and draining sexuality of its positive potency. Heyward argues that sexuality is actually one of the primary ways that people learn to value themselves and others:

---

21. In fact, she draws heavily upon Lorde and Nelson.
22. Plaskow, *Standing Again at Sinai,* 203.

As a western christian, I am interested in helping to lay to rest the pernicious dualisms between sex and God, sexuality and spirituality, body and spirit, and pleasure and goodness, which historically the church has used to dull the edges of human and divine experience. ... We have been stripped — spiritually, physically, emotionally and intellectually — of our capacities to delight in ourselves, one another, the creation, and its holy wellsprings.[23]

Therefore, as Heyward and others argue, the power and vitality of sexuality must be tapped even further, not restrained or repressed. Since sexuality is one of the primary ways people connect with one another, its healthy expression should be encouraged to flower. If feeling "alive" sexually enables people to demand joy, to expect justice, and to seek fullness of life, then this feeling should be encouraged.

Thus, feminist theologians of the erotic call themselves "sex-positive." At the very least, a sex-positive stance means repeatedly affirming that human sexuality is a deeply important good in human life. Sometimes these theologians claim sexuality to be sacred. The logic goes as follows: Because we must reject any dualism between the sexual and other dimensions of human life, we must also reject any association of sexuality with evil. If the sexual does not deserve to be cast aside as an inferior or "lower" aspect of human nature, then human sexuality should not only be celebrated but should also receive a central place in human experience. Therefore, sexuality is not finally separable from intellect, emotion, and even spirit because these are central, too. All dualisms should be replaced by the recognition of profound interconnection among the ways in which human persons mediate their existence in the world and before God. Plaskow perhaps characterizes this interconnection best:

[W]e cannot suppress our capacity for sexual feeling without suppressing our capacity for feeling more generally. If sexuality is one dimension of our ability to live passionately in the world, then in cutting off our sexual feelings, we diminish our overall power to feel, know, and value deeply. ... [I]nsofar as sexuality is an element in the embodiment that mediates our relation to reality, an aspect of the life energy that enables us to connect with others in creativity

---

23. Heyward, *Touching Our Strength*, 4.

and joy, sexuality is profoundly connected to spirituality, indeed is inseparable from it.[24]

In other words, sexuality is a significant avenue for knowing self, others, and God. If spirituality is, as the editors of *Sexuality and the Sacred* emphasize, a response of our whole beings to that which we find sacred, then this response includes our sexual being.[25] Thus, sexuality is sacred. Heyward even argues that through sexuality we participate in the divine. "We are embodied bearers of the erotic/God with one another, as she crosses over among us. The Sacred transcends us in our particularities, joining us together, erotically, as one body; in our sexual relationships as one flesh."[26]

Beyond calling sexuality sacred, feminist theologians of the erotic also understand themselves as visionaries of a positive sexuality. Marvin Ellison begins his book *Erotic Justice* with the quotation: "We must be prophets of a sex positive truth."[27] Likewise, sexual ethicist James Nelson tends not simply to affirm sexuality but to write about it in glorified, even mystical, terms: "Sexuality expresses the mystery of our creation as those who need to reach out for the physical and spiritual embrace of others."[28] While feminist theologians of the erotic are joined by many other contemporary thinkers who also affirm the goodness of human sexuality, they make affirmation of sexuality one of their central tasks. Moreover, they reverse the traditional equation of sexuality with immorality and equate sexuality instead with goodness — not even a neutral aspect of human life, which people might turn either to good or evil expression. To correct past emphases on evil, they tend to minimize any mention of sexual practices that might be evil, dangerous, or unhealthy, except to say that these are distortions of genuine sexuality. Acknowledgments of sexual evil (or even sexual banality) are always in reference to the way the meaning of sexuality has been twisted and perverted by tradition.

In summary, when feminist theologians of the erotic name the erotic as sensuality, they are invoking an alternative reality of pure, undistorted sensuality and sexuality. They are, in effect, claiming that the erotic is not only *not* the culprit of human sexual life but is its remedy. They are

---

24. Plaskow, *Standing Again at Sinai,* 196–97.
25. Nelson and Longfellow, *Sexuality and the Sacred,* xiv.
26. Heyward, *Touching Our Strength,* 128.
27. Larry J. Uhrig, *Sex Positive: A Gay Contribution to Sexual and Spiritual Union* (Boston: Alyson Publications, 1986), quoted in Ellison, *Erotic Justice,* 1.
28. Nelson, *Body Theology,* 22.

retrieving from the tradition the conviction that sexuality is an intensely powerful human drive, but exploiting this idea to create a new, much more positive theological meaning for the erotic. They claim that by having more confidence in our erotic, our embodied sensations and passions can become guiding forces for fulfillment. "The erotic — the sensual — [is] those physical, emotional, and psychic expressions of what is deepest and strongest and richest within each of us, being shared: the passions of love, in its deepest meanings."[29] Audre Lorde's speech, which is the prototype for the confident claims that characterize feminist theologies of the erotic, has inspired their insistence that all passions — physical, emotional, and psychic — lead to richness and fullness of life.

The Erotic as Wisdom

I have argued that feminist theologies of the erotic recover and reconstruct the classic notion of the erotic as a drive toward fullness of life. Sometimes the emphasis falls on the erotic *as* fullness; at other times, the erotic is emphasized as the vehicle for *reaching* fullness. That is, feminists aver that processes of feeling and intuition are themselves the erotic and also that they disclose the erotic. "The erotic" thus also becomes the name for a special mode of cognition, one used for reaching spiritual, interpersonal, and psychic fulfillment. This approach presents the erotic as wisdom.

Feminist theologians of the erotic claim that to get in touch with the erotic is to become wise to the truths about self, life, and world that will bring happiness and joy. The erotic as wisdom functions as a moral guide, revealing the true and the good. As Alexander Irwin observes:

> Feminists and womanists have also described Eros as a mode of cognition, a way of gaining deep and intimate knowledge of persons, things, and ideas. Erotic knowledge, they claim, is a form of wisdom that puts us in touch with the deepest levels of life itself.[30]

What distinguishes an erotic mode of cognition from other kinds of knowing? These writers call it "erotic knowing" or "erotic power" and liken it to intuition or other forms of nonrational cognition. Brock, for example, calls this way of knowing "knowing by heart," and for her it means a kind of intuitive awareness that is very different from ordinary

---

29. Lorde, "Uses of the Erotic," 56.
30. Irwin, *Eros toward the World,* 129.

reasoning or understanding. The mode of cognition people customarily use, she says, is detached, objective, and antithetical to passion. Knowing by heart, in contrast, is relational and subjective; feelings and passions are unabashedly engaged. There is great power, Brock claims, in this kind of erotic knowing. She gives an example of knowing by heart whereby objective, detached reasoning would not produce the same result as a more subjective and intimate cognition:

> For example, if I listen to a friend tell the story of a childhood molestation, her pain communicates itself vividly to me. But the pain I experience, triggered by hers, emerges from within me. It is not her pain, though it mirrors hers and enables me to take her pain into me. If I am oblivious to my own feelings and confuse mine with hers, I will experience my own pain through hers, making her uniqueness invisible. If I refuse my own feelings because I fear my own pain, my impassivity or my deflecting her pain by making it abstract or universal will reduce her presence to me. Maintaining my self-awareness, which allows my openness to her, allows me to respond in my own unique, creative way to her pain.[31]

Brock is saying that she can learn about, understand, and respond to her friend's memories better if she exploits rather than represses her own emotions and intuitions while listening. She claims that these nonrational avenues of wisdom enhance rather than detract from her knowing her friend's situation. Brock attributes the ability to respond uniquely and creatively to the erotic power flowing between teller and listener.

Usually, feminist theologians of the erotic talk about the erotic as wisdom in relation to discovering more positive things — joy, pleasure, and self-knowledge, to take some common examples. Perhaps the classic expression of the erotic as wisdom can be found in Lorde's metaphor of the "yes," a metaphor frequently borrowed by others: "We have been raised to fear the *yes* within ourselves, our deepest cravings."[32]

Saying "yes" is accessing some deep truth. Lorde and others claim that the erotic enables women (and men) to say "yes" to what they know, "deep down," to be good and true. Lorde argues that cravings which prove not to bring enhancement will be revealed as inauthentic and will

---

31. Brock, *Journeys by Heart*, 37.
32. Lorde, "Uses of the Erotic," 57.

naturally wither. The person who trusts her erotic, she implies, will be able simply to say "no" to such cravings. The desires will dissipate; they can be changed, presumably because while desires that enhance the self and those that harm both have staying power, only authentic desires will last after one discovers the erotic. The intuition, the assent — the "yes" — is reliable.

Feminist theologians of the erotic object that this way of knowing, if it is even acknowledged, tends to be discredited by most Westerners. They also note that we do not readily associate it with Eros. In everyday discourse, "the erotic" tends to connote only sex, or perhaps attraction to a lover. Therefore, we fail to appreciate other uses of the erotic, especially its ability to bring insight and wisdom. What prevents us from using the erotic as a source of knowledge? As one might expect, feminist theologians of the erotic argue that traditional beliefs in body-mind dualisms prevent us from gaining access to those sources of insight and wisdom that are not purely rational. We are reluctant to validate embodied and emotional forms of knowledge because we experience our bodies as separate from our minds and focus only on knowledge that comes through our minds. Negative attitudes toward the body, sex, and sensuality, that is, keep us from drawing upon nonrational sources of wisdom. Indeed, we readily assume that anything "known" through sensual means must be illicit. As evidence, feminist theologians of the erotic point to the classic conflation of the erotic with the pornographic. We presume that anything the body communicates to the mind is vaguely nasty. Therefore, we trivialize and ignore the genuine erotic and forfeit any wisdom it might mediate.

> The erotic has often been misnamed by men and used against women. It has been made into the confused, the trivial, the psychotic, the plasticized sensation. For this reason, we have often turned away from the exploration and consideration of the erotic as a source of power and information, confusing it with its opposite, the pornographic.[33]

Feminist theologians of the erotic nevertheless remain confident that erotic wisdom is a resource within all persons that simply needs to be tapped. They acknowledge that people must expand their ways of conceptualizing the erotic and grow accustomed to practicing erotic knowing, but think that once reconceptualization has occurred, erotic knowledge is

---

33. Lorde, "Uses of the Erotic," 54.

within everyone's grasp. Indeed, feminist theologians of the erotic insist
that the wisdom about how to attain fullness of life is inside every person,
simply awaiting the courageous individual who will unleash it.

Finally, in discourse about the erotic as wisdom, feminists frequently
claim that the erotic is a source of moral wisdom. In other words, they
call the erotic an ethical force, not just a personal resource. The erotic does
not simply liberate individuals but also changes the world. Irwin suggests
that this equating of the erotic with moral wisdom derives from the classic
feminist claim that "the personal is political":

> Of course, the idea that "the personal [including the sexual] is po-
> litical" has been something of a stock phrase in feminist circles for
> many years. Some religious feminist and womanist theorists, how-
> ever, have gone beyond the vagueness of the formula to make precise
> and challenging assertions about the political "uses of the erotic,"
> and about the nature of the connection between personal erotic
> experience and effective political and ethical engagement.[34]

Lorde, as we have seen, argued that the erotic could empower women
to engage in moral/political battles against patriarchy, racism, and other
forms of oppression. Feminist theologians of the erotic after her have
similarly claimed that the erotic is a source of inspiration and empowerment in political struggles. These theologians argue that once in touch
with the erotic, individuals become energized to join with one another to
challenge systems of domination and to work for justice. Ellison puts it
this way:

> Strong, morally principled eroticism gladdens people's hearts, minds,
> and souls, as well as their bodies. . . . In our sensuality, we find moral
> strength. This is a moral strength born of God, a strength to say
> "no" to injustice and to say an equally resounding "yes" to whatever
> promotes life, dignity, and hope throughout creation.[35]

In this guise, the feminist erotic functions as a resource for individual
and collective liberation and healing. In other words, for these theologians
the erotic is not only a powerful, sensual form of human love but also a
force for moral and political change. As Plaskow puts it, "If we repress

---

34. Irwin, *Eros toward the World*, 133.
35. Ellison, *Erotic Justice*, 120.

this knowledge because it also makes us sexually alive, then we repress the clarity and creative energy that is the basis of our capacity to envision and work for a more just social order."[36]

In summary, the erotic as wisdom is a cognitive process of gaining clarity and insight that motivates one to embrace the fullness of life which is within everyone's reach.

The Erotic as Relationality

According to feminist theologies of the erotic, one of the functions of the erotic as wisdom is to teach human beings how to be in "right relation." Heyward, for example, describes the erotic as our yearning to be in right relation, so that when we yield to the erotic, our love embodies right relationship. This approach leads to the last element I want to identify in feminist theological discourse about the erotic. In naming the erotic as a drive toward or desire for relationship, sometimes the erotic is identified with relationality itself.

What is relationality, and what does it mean to identify the erotic with it? Unfortunately, while feminist theologians of the erotic use the term frequently, they do not always indicate precisely what they mean by it. In general contemporary feminist discourse (apart from specific theologies of the erotic), however, two primary meanings of "relationality" are in use. On the one hand, the term sometimes (especially in philosophical discourse) signifies a feature of human nature typically contrasted with another feature, "autonomy." According to this meaning of the word, "relationality" simply indicates the fact that human beings are constituted as social creatures. In a functional and even ontological sense, we need one another to survive and to attain our life's goals. Moreover, we are significantly shaped by the social relationships of which we are a part.[37] On the other hand, "relationality" can also be taken to signify a feature or trait of particular personalities. According to this second meaning of the word, some individuals are more relational than others by virtue of the way their personalities have developed. Relational individuals are oriented toward the formation of interpersonal relationships. They make large emotional investments in relationships, spend a great deal of time

---

36. Plaskow, *Touching Our Strength,* 203.

37. Of course, a great deal of debate takes place over the extent to which the individual person is constituted by his or her relationships. The debate centers on the degree to which people are socially constituted versus the degree to which they can autonomously define themselves.

and energy on activities that will sustain them, and define themselves by
their relationships.

Many feminists (and nonfeminists) have linked this latter meaning of
relationality with the female personality. They believe that women are
fundamentally different from men in this regard.[38] They argue that since,
empirically, men typically devote less time to the creation and maintenance
of interpersonal relationships, the male personality must be "wired" differently. They point to evidence that men look less to relationships for
establishing emotional security and identity and more to the self. The female personality, in contrast, is responsible for the fact that many women
devote significant time and energy to relationships, use the level of a relationship as a barometer of their emotional security, and create personal
identity out of their relationships.[39] For these reasons, many feminists assume women to be more "relational" than men and "relationality" to be
a distinctly female trait.

The difference between these two meanings of the term "relationality"
is important to clarify, for it affects claims about the value of being relational. Individuals cannot become more relational in the first sense (they
simply are), and may or may not benefit from becoming more relational
in the second sense. In an article on the feminist debate over the ethics
of care, Jean Keller helpfully distinguishes relationality as a constitutive
feature of the human person from relationality as a trait.

> The care agent is thought to be relational not only in the gen-
> eral "socially constituted" sense — which all of us, even the most
> relationship-shy, share. Rather, the care agent is "relational" in the
> additional sense that one of the fundamental ways she conceives of
> herself and thinks about the world around her is in terms of the
> relationships in which she is involved.[40]

The feminist debate revolves, in part, around whether women being so
caring in this "additional sense" is valuable, or whether they are simply

---

38. Here the debate concerns the cause of this fundamental difference. Is relationality natural
or learned? Is it essential to being a woman or coincidental with the lives most women lead in a
way that leaves open the possibility of women being otherwise?

39. Some feminists, myself included, agree with many of these claims but do not think
they represent natural or essential differences between men and women. They rather represent
differences in psychosocial development.

40. Jean Keller, "Autonomy, Relationality, and Feminist Ethics," *Hypatia* 12, no. 2 (spring
1997): 158.

reinforcing constricting social constructions of womanhood by conceiving and displaying themselves this way. The same debate can bear upon feminist discourse about the erotic as relationality; shortly, I weigh in on the latter side of the debate. For now, however, let me return to the task of establishing what feminist theologians of the erotic mean when they say that the erotic is relationality.

Some feminist theologians of the erotic talk about the erotic as relationality when they want to celebrate the bonds of humanity present among all persons ("relationality" in the first sense described above). Brock, for instance, writes that "erotic power is the power of our primal interrelatedness."[41] In similar fashion, Heyward reminds her readers that "we come into this world connected, related, to one another — by blood and tissue, history, memory, culture, faith, joy, passion, violence, pain, and struggle."[42]

Other feminist theologians of the erotic explicitly equate the erotic with female relationality in the second, personality-oriented sense described above. Drawing upon the idea that Eros brings people together in intimate connection, and assuming that this is unequivocally a good thing, they conclude that the more intimacy and closeness a person is able to nurture in her relationships, the more erotic those relationships are. In other words, immersion in relationship is considered erotic, and an individual in touch with the erotic will exercise greater care, empathy, and attunement toward the other person. Another way to express this viewpoint is that erotic relationships are those wherein the "boundaries" between two partners are blurred, so close are they in identifying with each other. Inspired by the erotic, an individual is so aware of and attuned to the nuances of being in relationship with the other that she nearly forgets where she ends and the other begins. Feminist theologians of the erotic are not ignorant of feminist worries regarding women's loss of self in relation; however, a typical response is to deny that loss of self represents "true" eroticism. For example, Brock writes that "[an] open, interactive, self-expressiveness is different from either the need to impose our will upon the world or the need to lose ourselves in the feelings and needs of others. It is the root of intimacy and connection, and springs from and enhances our erotic power."[43]

---

41. Brock, *Journeys by Heart*, 26.
42. Heyward, *Touching Our Strength*, 192.
43. Brock, *Journeys by Heart*, 33.

Heyward and others (though not Brock) also identify relationality with women's sexuality and refer to women's actual sexual relationships as expressions of their "relational power." Heyward writes, for example, that in sexual relationships "we must be real with one another, really present: connected in our souls, the places in our bodyselves in which we know ourselves profoundly to be in relation."[44] This kind of discourse clarifies that becoming more, rather than less, relational is highly valued, and something that the individual can and should try to attain ("we *must* be...").

If in her discourse a theologian underscores the socially constituted nature of the human person and calls this nature the erotic, then she is simply expanding the definition of the erotic in yet another interesting, if unconventional, way. If, however, she implies that the erotic can only come to full fruition in relationships where the individual partners are fully "relational," this statement is tantamount to a claim that the flow of erotic passion depends on personalities that are not "relationship-shy" but, rather, oriented toward it. The more intense the relationality, the more erotic the relationship.

Feminist theologians of the erotic alternate between these meanings of the term. Heyward's warning against denying the power of the erotic gives us an example of such alternation:

> Locked within ourselves, holding secrets and denial, we embody not merely the fear of our relational possibilities; we also embody the rejection of the sacred ground of our being, which is none other than our power to connect. The fear of mutuality is the fear of our intrinsic interrelatedness, the fact that literally I am nobody without you.[45]

In this passage, Heyward equates the erotic not only with virtues like honesty, but also with personality traits like openness, and still again with a basic interrelatedness of human existence. She blurs these different meanings; knowing whether she is affirming human sociality or specific moral behaviors becomes difficult. One could also describe what Heyward is doing as conflating the feature of relationality with the norm of mutuality.

Tying the erotic too closely to relationality can be dangerous, and the reasons for this concern become clear as the book progresses. Suffice it to

---

44. Heyward, *Touching Our Strength,* 33 and 131, respectively.
45. Heyward, *Touching Our Strength,* 21.

say now that, especially in their discourse about the erotic as relationality, feminist theologians of the erotic depart the farthest from traditional understandings of Eros and also make the most problematic claims with regard to feminism. Feminist theologians of the erotic are wise to insist that human persons are not entirely self-reliant creatures and that the relational bonds we form give our lives tremendous meaning. They do a service to sexual ethicists and others by recovering the notion that to flourish as human beings, individuals in relationship need sometimes to yield to the other and to practice greater care and sympathy. But this discourse needs to be balanced by a discourse that affirms *not* always yielding to others. Sometimes the bonds of relationship can be too alluring and must be resisted; nowhere is this more evident than in sexual relationships. (For one partner to believe that she is "nobody" without the other is dangerous in a sexual context because such a belief makes her vulnerable to tolerating abuse.) Therefore, at least when working toward an ethics of sexuality for adolescents, feminists must continue to approve individualism, separateness, and self-assertion, and even teach the next generation how to develop them. In erotic relationships, identification with the other must always be balanced by assertion of self. This approach in no way disregards the socially constituted nature of human life. In fact, only by recognizing why some people, especially girls and women, are constituted as relational can we fully appreciate the need not to glorify and idealize "relationality."

Celebrations of the erotic as love, as sensuality, as wisdom, and as relationality are hallmarks of the feminist theological discourse about the erotic that is gaining an ever wider audience. These categories do not exhaust the meanings of the erotic for these theologians; their collective body of work on sexuality, gender, and love is too rich and diverse. But understanding these four ways of talking about Eros gives us a good introduction to this movement to recover the erotic within theology and ethics. The writers I am calling feminist theologians of the erotic are not only recovering some of the best in the Western tradition but critiquing that tradition at the same time and therefore trying to move it forward. They are even responding to earlier feminist discourses about women and women's sexuality. In summary, feminist theologies of the erotic challenge all who would think anew about gender and sexuality to identify the negative ideologies of the erotic we have inherited from our past and replace them with new ones. These theologies remind us of the many ways human persons have been taught to deny and despise erotic passion, especially sexual passion. They tirelessly argue that human beings need to have more confidence in the power of the erotic, for it is nothing to fear and something to rely on. We turn now to five representative theologians to see how these claims are worked out in more detail in particular texts.

An Appraisal of Feminist Theologies of the Erotic

Looking at representative texts helps a study of feminist theologies of the erotic. The texts selected for this discussion are Audre Lorde's "Uses of the Erotic: The Erotic as Power," Carter Heyward's *Touching Our Strength: The Erotic as Power and the Love of God,* Rita Nakashima Brock's *Journeys by Heart: A Christology of Erotic Power,* Anne Bathurst Gilson's *Eros Breaking Free: Interpreting Sexual Theo-Ethics,* and Marvin Ellison's *Erotic Justice: A Liberating Ethic of Sexuality.* These texts hold most, if not all, of the claims discussed above in common. They seek to recover the erotic by redefining and strengthening an erotic discourse, and they all tie this discourse implicitly, if not explicitly, to sexual ethics. In the analyses that follow, I further clarify my own points of disagreement with these theologians. I argue that feminist theologies of the erotic helpfully link moral problems in sexuality to impoverished estimations of what is possible in human flourishing, but they unhelpfully assume that an adequate remedy to these problems lies in simple naming or reclaiming of the erotic. If feminist theologians of the erotic are correct to remind us that we need to have more confidence in erotic passions, they are mistaken to place too much confidence in the erotic themselves. The erotic is not always the solution they suppose. Often, the erotic is the problem.

Audre Lorde

As indicated above, Audre Lorde's essay, "Uses of the Erotic: The Erotic as Power," was one of the first, and remains one of the most significant, feminist articulations of confidence in the erotic. While Lorde did not identify herself as a religious, let alone theological, thinker, this work nevertheless became a point of departure for many feminist theologians.[46] In her essay, Lorde never offers one definitive meaning of the erotic,

---

46. One theologian has called it a "touchstone" for feminist and womanist theologians. Another calls it "virtually canonical." See Irwin, *Eros toward the World,* 124, and Kathleen Sands, "Uses of the Thea(o)logian," 11, respectively.

but rather describes it in many different ways. In terms of the typology above, Lorde most often writes about the erotic as sensuality and wisdom. She starts by saying that the erotic is "a resource within each of us that lies in a deeply female and spiritual plane, firmly rooted in the power of our unexpressed or unrecognized feeling."[47] According to Lorde, the erotic is like an untapped well within each woman, long suppressed but powerful. If women were to overcome their fear and suspicion of strong feelings, they would be greatly empowered. By recognizing, reclaiming, and affirming this source within themselves, women would be liberated to realize a potential they are generally not now actualizing.

Perhaps the best way to capture the meaning of Lorde's erotic is to cite her own comparison of the erotic to energy.

> When I speak of the erotic, then, I speak of it as an assertion of the lifeforce of women; of that creative energy empowered, the knowledge and use of which we are now reclaiming in our language, our history, our dancing, our loving, our work, our lives.[48]

In effect, Lorde is saying that the erotic is like a generic force with potential to suffuse and inform everything a woman does. Not limited to sexual energy, but still somehow embodied and sensual, Lorde's erotic enlivens all manner of ordinary activities, energizing everything from "dancing, building a bookcase, writing a poem, [to] examining an idea."[49] The erotic transforms the ordinary into the extraordinary, and like physical or chemical energy, may take different forms but is always conserved and therefore always available to be tapped.

How does Lorde explain the fact that few women share her understanding of the erotic? Does the erotic mean something different for them, or are they simply missing something? What explains the suffering many women experience and associate with erotic passions? Lorde responds that women suffer under mischaracterizations and abuses of the erotic that an androcentric culture forces upon them. For example, women are susceptible to distorted thinking when their culture persuades them that the erotic is the same as the pornographic. They too often accept the conflation of sex and violence that pornography portrays as normal and even normative, despite disproportionately suffering from this conflation when victimized

---

47. Lorde, "Uses of the Erotic," 53.
48. Lorde, "Uses of the Erotic," 55.
49. Lorde, "Uses of the Erotic," 56–57.

by sexual violence. The erotic itself is abused when denied, and in this way, women are abused, according to Lorde. She gives the example of one partner taking advantage of the other's feelings. Taking advantage of another in the name of relationship is the opposite of eroticism; it is not an expression of the genuine erotic. Lorde also mentions the way people too often satisfy their erotic feelings in destructive ways because they have no other outlet — they engage in "certain proscribed erotic comings together." These acts, she argues, are just an example of corrupted erotic needs.[50]

Lorde thus responds to the fact of sexual misery and confusion by explaining it as the erotic gone bad — denied, distorted, corrupted. In its true (meaning for Lorde unsullied) state, the erotic is always good. Passions or desires only become problematic when people mischaracterize, ignore, or suppress them. Accordingly, the answer to these problems would be placing greater trust in the erotic:

> As women we have come to distrust that power which rises from our deepest and nonrational knowledge. We have been warned against it all our lives by the male world. . . . But the erotic offers a well of replenishing and provocative force to the woman who does not fear its revelation, nor succumb to the belief that sensation is enough.[51]

For Lorde, then, the most important remedies to misery and confusion lie in acts of self-empowerment by trusting the erotic within. If women can only characterize the erotic properly, attend to its demands, and release its potency, she says, they can overcome most of the problems associated with it. "Once we know the extent to which we are capable of feeling that sense of satisfaction and completion, we can then observe which of our various life endeavors bring us closest to that fullness."[52] This statement appears to imply that women who cannot overcome their problems cannot do so because of their own internal obstacles. If the erotic works "for the woman who *does not fear* its revelation, *nor succumb* to the belief that sensation is enough," then the woman with enough courage will prevail. The erotic will be liberated in her, but not necessarily in those who are still afraid or confused because their social location keeps them disempowered.

---

50. Lorde, "Uses of the Erotic," 59.
51. Lorde, "Uses of the Erotic," 53–54.
52. Lorde, "Uses of the Erotic," 54–55.

Lorde seems even to be saying that some women are doomed never to recover their erotic while others will be successful. She offers herself as an example: As a black lesbian feminist, she is no stranger to others' attempts to repress her passions and is therefore practiced in resisting repression. She says, however, that the "erotic charge" she feels "is not easily shared by women who continue to operate under an exclusively european-american male tradition."[53] Lorde may simply be saying here that oppression makes one especially perceptive about the effects of power, but that women consciously choose under which traditions they will operate is also strongly suggested. This approach seems somehow incoherent. She cannot easily argue that the erotic provides a resource for political critique and then omit from this project people who live under the politics that needs critiquing. Lorde compounds this problem by leveling an implicit criticism against women who do not demand erotic empowerment from themselves: "But giving in to the fear of feeling and working to capacity is a luxury only the unintentional can afford, and the unintentional are those who do not wish to guide their own destinies."[54] Lorde seems not to recognize that "unintentional" fear and passivity are the exact things constraining some women.

Lorde's analysis also falters in a second way: her descriptions of the erotic contain certain unrecognized assumptions regarding gender. She identifies the erotic closely with female experience but does not explain what is female about it, or whether girls' and women's sensitivity to it is always a good thing. One wonders whether many men would recognize the erotic as a force that connects all their physical, emotional, and spiritual desires in the way Lorde describes — or whether Lorde thinks they would. Perhaps uniting all these desires under one force simply reflects women's attempt to connect their love for their work with their love for persons with their love for the earth to attend to all their needs and desires (and those of others) simultaneously without tension. If so, experiencing the erotic as a lifeforce is only derivatively a female experience. In addition, Lorde fails to recognize that there are men who do not "operate under an exclusively european-american male tradition" and who might share the erotic charge of resisting oppression. She blithely identifies the male erotic

---

53. Lorde, "Uses of the Erotic," 59.
54. Lorde, "Uses of the Erotic," 54.

with patriarchy and thus ignores men, such as gay men, whose experience may be closer to her own as a lesbian. In other words, even though many of Lorde's descriptions of the erotic are couched in broad and universal language, they are not, in the end, inclusive.

Several difficulties attend Lorde's approach to the erotic, especially insofar as it carries implications for sexual ethics. First, Lorde's confidence in the erotic appears overly sanguine. She cannot account for the complexities and ironies of erotic desiring. For most people, once they discover what satisfies them, they cannot continue simply and consistently to achieve the same satisfaction and fullness. The meaning of erotic passion is not stable, and its interpretation is not so simple. Sometimes, too, changing one's erotic response can be tremendously difficult. A deep and pervasive interest in pornography, to use Lorde's example, cannot simply be overcome, as Lorde suggests, by recalling the true meaning of the erotic. The erotic spell of pornography cannot be broken simply by asserting more "lifeforce." The reasons people find it compelling are too complex for such a simplistic solution. In other words, critiquing our culture's prevailing ideologies about what is and is not erotic and then asserting an alternative one are not enough. People who hope for change must also analyze how certain ideologies about the erotic seep in and take hold within the individual psyche, affecting even those who "know better."

Second, Lorde cannot account for how the person in whom the erotic is distorted can be the same person to release it. How does an individual come to realize that her erotic potential needs emancipation in the first place? How can the erotic be both continually repressed and serve as a liberating source? Lorde's erotic just somehow seems to liberate itself. In other words, her discourse about the erotic is not only overly sanguine but also potentially contradictory.

I have probably leveled too much criticism for such a short essay as "Uses of the Erotic." I acknowledge that this piece was written as a speech and was presumably intended to be more inspirational than analytical. Because Lorde was primarily a poet and essayist, perhaps expecting this speech of hers to resolve so many practical and theoretical problems about the erotic is unfair. Nevertheless, this short essay has had profound influence and has won much praise. Insofar as feminist theologians of the erotic have relied on its inspiration in their own work, the level of criticism is fair. Feminists who have given much more sustained attention to these issues still display the same contradictions, so pointing them out becomes important.

To cultivate the germinal ideas in Lorde's essay, one would need, I think, to examine the ways in which reclaiming the erotic is a social as well as individual task. The erotic will not be liberated unless the individual is liberated first. Individual women alone cannot release their own erotic in any way that would amount to a significant recovery. Its socially and culturally produced meanings are too deeply internalized. The reasons that girls and women are fearful of the erotic and find so little erotic satisfaction is not that they have not yet had any erotic experiences to know about, but because they have. Experiencing erotic passion scares and perplexes many girls. It may evoke a certain power and intensity, and even satisfaction, but girls often choose to ignore this power. As I demonstrate later, many adolescent girls confront a conflict between knowing and yet not knowing about their erotic feelings. They resolve this conflict by disavowing their own feelings and knowledge because this resolution appears to be their only choice as girls. In other words, girls are not free because they are *girls,* not because they have not discovered their erotic. Liberation from gender injustice — the injustice of having too few options besides disavowing the self — is really at the root of any erotic liberation. Creating other options will be an ongoing, collective task.

In summary, while we can appreciate the need for a dramatically different discourse about the erotic, Lorde's discourse runs the risks of being overly optimistic, contradictory, and — perhaps inadvertently — of burdening the people most oppressed with responsibility for their own liberation. Lorde's influential essay has helped many to see the way Western culture has woefully understood erotic passion. She named the misery many women were feeling and pointed many women toward the joy erotic energy could bring. But to weave a discourse about adolescent sexuality on Lorde's loom would be to smooth over too much of its subtle, ironic, tragic, and variegated texture.

Carter Heyward

As a religious feminist, Carter Heyward applies many of Lorde's insights to her own reworking of Christian themes, especially that of Christian love. She attempts to construct a comprehensive theology of the erotic in her book, *Touching Our Strength: The Erotic as Power and the Love of God.* This book represents the most thorough articulation to date of feminist discourse about the erotic. Heyward begins by declaring the erotic "foundational to both sexual pleasure and play and to justice-making," thereby continuing Lorde's commitment to naming as "erotic" a wide variety of passions and activities.[55] She tends to maintain a closer connection than Lorde between passion that is religious or spiritual and that which is specifically sexual. Her theological argument weaves through discussions of essentialism, heterosexism, abuse, redemption, and ethics. The main thread running through it all is the need to move away from a dualistic, alienated, and alienating sexuality into mutuality and right relation. People can achieve right relation, argues Heyward, when they discover that true erotic power is the sacred power that operates between and among persons.

Like Lorde, Heyward's rhetoric about the erotic is quite sanguine. That Heyward's defense of the erotic is often compelling cannot be denied. Her images are very appealing, and the reader wishes to agree that they capture some true essence of the erotic.

> Basking together in a warm field can be a highly eroticized experience for those delighted by the mingling of sex and the natural world. Opening me to wildflowers, sun, and to the one beside me, the power of the erotic draws me out, unfolding me more and more, to my partner and our meadowed bed. Our boundaries become fluid, light, easy to move through into one another's bodyselves.[56]

Moreover, Heyward's descriptions consistently deconstruct any rigid differences between the erotic and the sacred. She does this by blurring distinctions between physical and spiritual sensations; for example, she refers to "yearning" and "transcendence" as simultaneously physical and spiritual.

> The erotic is our most fully embodied experience of the love of God. As such, it is the source of our capacity for transcendence, the "crossing over" among ourselves, making connections between ourselves in relation. The erotic is the divine Spirit's yearning, which is our most fully embodied experience of God as love.[57]

---

55. Heyward, *Touching Our Strength*, 3.
56. Heyward, *Touching Our Strength*, 113.
57. Heyward, *Touching Our Strength*, 99.

Strong reasons exist to appreciate the connections Heyward is trying to draw. For too long, erotic passions have been set in opposition to spiritual ones. Sexual desire and pleasure in particular (especially women's) have been severely discredited as valid manifestations of human vitality and love. Moreover, sexuality is one of the most important avenues for human persons to experience transcendence. Sexual mergence with another yields a special opportunity to transcend the boundaries of the self and grow in awareness and love, because sex provides those moments of bliss, of awakening to oneself through losing oneself, that too often we rarely feel otherwise. Affirming the power and importance of sexuality in this way is tremendously important.

And yet, ironically, Heyward overreaches. Simply put, sex is not always blissful, and "erotic" does not always evoke delightful, warm basking. Sometimes pleasure does not come in this package, and sometimes sex is terribly banal. Quite simply, not all instances of erotic desire bring about blissful transcendence of self. Heyward has identified something genuine, but not universal. "There is a truth here," as Barbara Hilkert Andolsen says, but one that most of us "only sometimes know."[58] Or, as Kathleen Sands says more bluntly: "Carter Heyward may be luckier than I and my friends, but from what I hear there are inevitable and sometimes serious points of tension between relational commitment and the pursuit of sexual pleasure."[59] In an attempt to affirm that we can express our love of others and of God through embodied erotic experience, Heyward ends up romanticizing women's experience of the erotic. She risks drawing an unreal, overly glorified picture of erotic experience.

Furthermore, the loss of boundaries can be destructive as well as positive in sexual experience. Perhaps all adults seek in sex a sense of infantile union with another, but when this desire is associated with a tendency to lose a sense of self more generally, such a desire can be harmful. This tendency, as we shall see, often typifies girls' experience of romance and sex, and to no good end. Heyward's "crossing over" may become no more than a willingness to submerge the self in connection.

Heyward chiefly writes about the erotic as relationality, though it is always an embodied, sensual power for her. Sexual/erotic pleasure is a

---

58. Barbara Hilkert Andolsen, "Whose Sexuality? Whose Tradition? Women, Experience, and Roman Catholic Sexual Ethics," in *Religion and Sexual Health*, ed. Ronald M. Green (Boston: Kluwer Academic Publishers, 1992), 73.

59. Sands, "Uses of the Thea(o)logian," 21.

relational power that connects one with self, other, and God. Indeed, Heyward asserts that the very presence of the divine is manifest in our human capacity for relationality. Relationality is divine. God is the power to be relational. In the glossary to her book, she defines God this way: "God is our power in mutual relation. . . . By this power, we god."[60]

Which sense of "relationality" Heyward means here is open to interpretation. Perhaps she simply intends to remind us that we are always constituted in some basic sense as "friends" of one another, or to put it theologically, that the movement of ongoing connection is the imprint of the divine on the human. But her context is almost always that of special relationships. For Heyward, particular, intimate relationships are at least the paradigmatic manifestation of "relational power." With specific friends and lovers we express our "true" relationality. Hence, "relationality" seems to mean the actual exercise of being in relationship, despite the way she habitually uses ontological language.

Heyward is careful to distinguish "right relation" from "wrong relation." In other words, she does not uncritically endorse relationality, but more specifically endorses being in right relation. Upon examination, however, Heyward turns out to have few non-self-referential ways to identify right relation and to distinguish it from wrong relation. Right relation is true relation, which is discerned when persons are empowered to be relational. Wrong relation is untrue — "perverse" — and becomes evident when persons are not "themselves," a condition itself caused primarily by their failure to embrace their relationality. These definitions are circular or self-referential, and what right relation means apart from becoming more relational and wrong relation apart from not being relational is unclear. Heyward's language is frequently imprecise this way; for example, she writes elsewhere, "Our power in relation is being shaped in the matrix of each relational self who is true to herself as relational."[61]

According to Heyward's definitions, right relation is true and wrong relation is untrue. She effectively equates the right/good with truth and wrong/evil with falsity. Such an equation can be philosophically problematic, for it effectively suggests that evil is not real and thus always runs the risk of letting it go unexplained.

This approach becomes especially problematic when treating erotic pas-

---

60. Heyward, *Touching Our Strength,* 188–90.
61. Heyward, *Touching Our Strength,* 33.

sion. If the erotic is constructed as relationality, it, too, is essentially good. Like Lorde, Heyward maintains that the only time the erotic fails to lead one to that which is true/good is when one does not believe in it. Problems associated with erotic passion stem from lack of understanding and faith. Both Lorde and Heyward insist that the genuine nature of the erotic is good, and only when people's confidence falters, or their minds are stolen from them by people who would distort erotic power, does it go bad. This argument is as problematic in Heyward as in Lorde, leaving "bad" (unhealthy, excessive, or perverted) desires unexplained. Within the theory, they are awkward leftovers, simply failures in faith and freedom. They become anomalies of the erotic, rather than unfortunate but real and persistent desires to which persons are sometimes prone. As Kathleen Sands writes of the same religious feminists I critique:

> The good is established by true understanding rather than by actualization. Evil or deviance, while declared anomalous, are not actually prevented from *being*. They are only prevented from *being acknowledged* as what they are. . . . When it comes to injustice within sex itself we often speak as if we were dealing with an intellectual rather than a political and social problem. . . .[62]

Heyward might respond by saying that a woman who passively submits to seduction (a "bad" erotic desire), for example, is not being "true" to her erotic power-in-relation. But this argument assumes that an erotic somewhere "inside" or "out there" is present — a wonderful erotic that *exists* in some real yet invisible place — that this woman has not yet tapped. A more adequate analysis, although admittedly a less appealing one, might be that this woman finds submitting to seduction erotic. (This feeling would not necessarily be in contrast to her also finding it troubling to want to submit.) The theoretical challenge would be to figure out how submission-as-erotic is constructed in the first place as desirable for her and for other women. For transformation to occur, submission would have to

---

62. "Uses of the Thea(o)logian," 8. I am indebted to Sands for pointing out the philosophical pitfalls in the thinking of Heyward and other religious feminists. The denial of any difference between the true and the good poses especially serious difficulties when trying to account theologically for sexual abuse, assault, and coercion, which are the subject of Sands's concern as one interested in questions of theodicy. She argues that these abuses cannot be denied as true instances of sexual passion, even if they are evil. Sands suggests that sexuality be treated theologically as an instance of tragedy, an element of human life containing both good and evil.

become unerotic, undesirable, which in turn would require a fundamental transformation in constructions of gender, power, and sexuality.

We must therefore hesitate before relying too greatly on. Heyward's conception of the erotic as relationality, especially with respect to sexuality. Pitfalls exist in praising relationality too highly, and serious problems emerge in treating it as a norm for sexual relationship. Some of these same issues become apparent in examining the very different work of Rita Nakashima Brock.

Rita Nakashima Brock

The meaning of erotic in Rita Nakashima Brock's *Journeys by Heart: A Christology of Erotic Power* is significantly different from that in Lorde's and Heyward's discourses, even though she draws approvingly from their work. Unlike Heyward, for Brock the erotic is only dimly related to physical sexuality. In contrast to Lorde, Brock's definition of the erotic is somewhat narrower; Brock does not have in mind some energizing passion for whatever is empowering. Rather, Brock's notion of the erotic remains consistently tied to relationality. She speaks of it as Feminist Eros and defines it as "far more than sexuality, passion, or an intellectual or spiritual quest for ideal beauty. Feminist Eros is grounded in the relational lives of women and in a critical, self-aware consciousness that unites the psychological and political spheres of life, binding love with power."[63] Indeed, when Brock writes about the erotic, she is writing about an ontological reality, a fundamental constituent of human life. The erotic is relationality, or, as Brock often puts it, the human capacity for "connection." "Connection is the basic power of all existence, the root of life. The power of being/becoming is erotic power."[64]

Erotic power, for Brock, is the deep human drive to form and to sustain bonds with others. Brock brings psychoanalytic theory, especially Alice Miller's and Nancy Chodorow's theories of object relations, to her discourse. Thus, in Brock's work, the meaning of "relational" is a psychoanalytic one, and her claims about the erotic as relationality must also be interpreted as such. To put it simply, Brock's understanding of erotic power starts with the basic premise of object relations theory: Human persons are fundamentally object-seeking. Drawing upon Miller, she argues

---

63. Brock, *Journeys by Heart*, 26.
64. Brock, *Journeys by Heart*, 41.

that the self is produced out of relationships with other objects (meaning the self's symbolic psychic representations of other persons): "The self is an achievement of our relationality, structured in our existence from birth, as our ever-changing physical existence is a structured reality at birth."[65] Brock then links this technical, psychoanalytic view of the self to the feminist discourse about the erotic, and the result is a hybrid of the two. Erotic power becomes the fundamental movement of human persons to connect with others.

> The erotic is the basis of being itself as the power of relationship, and all existence comes to be by virtue of connectedness, from atoms to the cosmos. Erotic power is the fundamental power of existence-as-a-relational-process. . . . We are born in it as we are born in the physical structures of the universe.[66]

As a hybrid, Brock's discourse about the erotic as relationality does not distinguish between the two meanings of relationality discussed earlier. When she talks about erotic power, she conflates two meanings — ontological reality and female personality trait. For example, she makes the following statements: "Erotic power, as it creates and connects hearts, involves the whole person in relationships of self-awareness, vulnerability, openness, and caring." "Erotic power grounds the concreteness of our experiences of empathy, passion, creativity, sensuality, and beauty."[67] As these statements demonstrate, Brock aligns erotic power with concrete experiences of passion and creativity in relationship, with qualities like openness and vulnerability, and with attitudes like care and empathy. In such a discourse, erotic power becomes not just an underlying constituent of human existence, but a set of specific and even normative qualities. But these qualities have typically characterized women's lives. The effect is that Brock's "erotic power" comes dangerously close to the typical female profile of relationality.

At one point, Brock seems to sense the danger. She is aware that the association of femininity with relationality is a construction:

> Females develop a sense of identity by connection to and dependence on others and pay closer attention to their day-to-day environment.

65. Brock, *Journeys by Heart*, 17.
66. Brock, *Journeys by Heart*, 41.
67. Brock, *Journeys by Heart*, 26.

Feminine identity feels itself incomplete without a complex of relationships of differing kinds. The feminine self avoids open conflict
and competition and feels herself confirmed in the capacity to nurture others — to be attuned to and to seek to meet the needs of
others.[68]

Yet in her own constructive statements about the erotic, she uses strik-
ingly similar language. She talks about "connection" and "relationship"
when she is describing her vision of erotic power. Therefore, like Lorde's,
Brock's erotic is infused with unacknowledged gendered assumptions.

If the erotic becomes too similar to the female trait of relationality, a
fair question to ask is whether a call for the recovery of the erotic can
provide a necessary critique of relationality. Brock does not sufficiently
distinguish her ontological claim that all people need and thrive on connection from her psychological observation that women's sense of self
lies largely *in* connection. She conflates the notions of ontological connectedness and the psychological need to maintain relational bonds. She
thus ends up exaggerating the need for women to recover their original connected and relational natures. Whether this nature is original for
women or a construction that might be politically necessary to challenge,
however, is the crucial prior question. Other feminist theorists, including
object relations theorists, struggle with this question, thus tempering the
confidence with which they claim to know what women want and need.
Brock's theory could use a dose of their skepticism.

Anne Bathurst Gilson

Anne Bathurst Gilson's *Eros Breaking Free* initially seems to promise a theology of the erotic that corrects some problems that the other theologies
present. In this book Gilson offers some critique of the feminist theologians to whom she is indebted (Lorde, Heyward, and Brock, as well as
Sheila Briggs) and thus attempts to advance their discourse. She puts her
finger on the dilemma facing a feminist who wishes to affirm earlier work
and yet challenge it as well:

I understand the reluctance of feminist theologians — who are just
beginning to reclaim, re-define, and reconstruct Eros — to address
aspects of Eros that are not empowering and, in fact, have damaged

---

68. Brock, *Journeys by Heart*, 15.

women and children. Some feminist liberation theo-ethicists hesitate
to engage the issue of a distorted and violent Eros, the issue of an
abusive sexuality, because of the fear that doing so would evoke "I
told you so" responses from those who would keep tighter reigns on
Eros and sexuality. But by giving into that fear, feminist liberation
theo-ethicists risk the power of the unspoken becoming greater than
the power of the spoken.[69]

Gilson notes that the "unspoken" — the disempowering and damaging potential of Eros — is difficult to articulate without reverting to the language
of denigration that previously characterized Christian attitudes toward the
erotic. But she insists that the answer to this difficulty is not simply to glorify the erotic; the potentially negative paths that Eros travels along must
be acknowledged alongside the positive ones. She therefore identifies some
of the difficult questions that a thoroughly affirmative view of the erotic
obscures:

New questions are emerging as to what ethical guidelines are needed
in what situations. . . . Are there any "controls" to be put on sexuality?
If so, what are they, and who decides what they are? What does
mutuality actually mean, practically speaking, in our day-to-day lives?
How do we struggle to move toward mutuality relationally?[70]

In asking these questions, Gilson acknowledges that sexual ethics needs
to move in some new direction, neither imposing "tighter reigns" on erotic
experience nor succumbing to normlessness. She also acknowledges that
mutuality is itself a struggle and therefore cannot serve as an ethical guide-
line. She suggests that simply redefining the erotic in terms of mutuality
or relationality and supposing that, if the erotic is liberated, our day-to-
day interactions will reach mutuality is not enough. For this approach
to become an actual norm for sexual life, we need something more than
the emancipation of Eros. Unfortunately, Gilson's book (entitled, after
all, *Eros Breaking Free*) does not provide it. She leaves many of her own
questions unanswered. She continues, along with the feminists she re-
views, to be primarily concerned with how to wrest the erotic free of
its former taboos. With other feminist theologians of the erotic, Gilson

69. Gilson, *Eros Breaking Free*, 87–88.
70. Gilson, *Eros Breaking Free*, 83–84.

unabashedly admits tremendous faith in the power of the erotic.[71] Like Lorde, Heyward, and Brock, Gilson believes the erotic succeeds because and when it is true and right; and despite her acknowledgment that it sometimes fails to bring fullness of life, Gilson argues that, when set free, the erotic generates its own moral norms. In particular, she maintains that the erotic naturally moves toward love of self, God, and other and away from alienation and disintegration.

In short, Gilson's theology does not succeed in avoiding the problems that plague feminist theologies of the erotic. Though she hints at some of the work that still needs to be done before feminists can develop an adequate sexual ethic, her book does not deliver on its initial promises and does not represent a significant departure from earlier ideas. To be fair, Gilson's book is more concerned with ecclesiology than theory, as she largely treats sexual ethics from the perspective of church policies and practices. Accordingly, she does not presume to answer the above questions, but instead outlines strategies that will be useful to others in answering them. For example, she suggests that more contexts be created within the church for personal, forthright discussions about sexuality among people whose sexual histories differ because of their different social locations.

Yet Gilson claims to be making contributions to a more liberated theological ethic of sexuality. Her two main contributions are, first, a suggestion that we envision God as sexual, and, second, the theory that fear lies in the way of truly liberated sexuality. She maintains that women can overcome fear through sufficient self-empowerment. She argues that creating genuinely mutual sexuality involves mustering up what it takes — primarily, better communication — to move beyond damaging patterns of relationship. Women can do these things, she says, if they talk with each other and their partners and learn to trust their bodies. She acknowledges that different people fear different things sexually and that many women in particular especially fear losing their connections with others. She does not, however, go on to analyze women's predisposition to fearfulness of this sort and, more importantly, she does not link this insight about connectedness to women's unliberated sexuality. She does not realize that in their fearful attempts to prevent the loss of connection, women actually disavow themselves, a process that itself alienates and disintegrates.

---

71. Gilson, *Eros Breaking Free,* 109. Gilson explicitly defends her faith in the erotic against Sands's skepticism.

In summary, like other feminist theologians of the erotic, Gilson seems uncognizant of the notion that the erotic cannot empower women if they remain focused on the individual and conscious level. What women need instead is to engage in systemic critical theory about the sociology, psychology, and politics of their disempowerment.

Marvin Ellison

Marvin Ellison is one theologian who *has* developed a systematic sexual ethic; he offers the fullest effort to date to develop an ethic that takes seriously both erotic passion and justice. His work is therefore in some ways the most promising of the writers we have considered. Ellison identifies himself as a social ethicist "in sync with progressive people of all genders, classes, and colors who, like myself, have committed their life energy to confronting oppression . . ."[72] and is therefore included here as a feminist writer. Ellison does not focus on the erotic per se in the same way that other feminist theologians of the erotic do, but he shares many of the same premises, draws approvingly upon their work, and sees himself as carrying that work forward.

Erotic Justice: A Liberating Ethic of Sexuality is Ellison's visionary statement. In it he calls for a wholesale reconstruction of a Christian ethic of sexuality. This new approach will primarily come about, he argues, through dismantling Christianity's legacy of sex-negativity along with its indirect support of sexism, racism, and homophobia. Ellison is attentive to current theories of sexuality and gender and therefore avoids some of the naiveté that characterizes earlier writers. He also wisely regards sexuality as a social and political issue and resists any simple celebration of the erotic as we know it. Nevertheless, his project does not go far enough in expanding or supplementing other feminist theologies of the erotic. Despite his insights into the social and political dimensions of sexuality, his proposals still place sexuality within an individualistic framework. He does not critically analyze it as a product of power and gender. In the end, he remains gripped by the construct of Eros-as-personal-resource just as are other feminist theologians of the erotic.

Ellison begins by asserting that sexuality and the erotic are dialectically related to the social and political order. (Ellison would add "the erotic as politics" to our typology of constructions of the erotic.) The meaning of

---

72. Ellison, *Erotic Justice*, 3.

sexuality varies from culture to culture and from era to era, and sexuality is therefore a plastic thing, not formed as an essential given. In addition to arguing for the plasticity of sexuality, Ellison argues that sexuality is captured by forces outside itself. For Ellison, what it means for sexuality to be "socially constructed" is that sexual injustice is but one manifestation of a larger interconnected web of social injustices. "The bad news, in evidence everywhere, is that human sexuality is distorted by various forms of social oppression."[73] Ellison is also fond of saying that sexism, racism, and other injustices are felt at the somatic level. People literally embody the effects of social injustice.

In explaining how this works, Ellison draws briefly upon the theory of John Gagnon and William Simon, two sociologists whose work on sexuality has been widely influential and supportive of social constructionism. Briefly, Gagnon and Simon argue that society constructs codes and scripts that people learn to obey in order to conform. This learning occurs at a barely conscious level, so subtle yet powerful is the societal encoding and scripting. Included in this process are cultural codes about sexuality, that is, unspoken rules that dictate what kind of sexual behaviors and attitudes are acceptable for people of different genders, races, and so on. People conform to models of sexuality that they and others perceive to be appropriate to who they are.[74] Ellison draws upon Gagnon and Simon to argue that one of the most powerful and pervasive sexual codes in our society is one that gives people with greater power permission to practice sex that controls and belittles those with lesser power. In this way, control and domination become sexy; they become eroticized. People accept the equation of Eros with this kind of power, and their behavior comes to reflect it. (Ellison echoes Lorde here.) In effect, they play the part given to them and, in their so doing, the "part" becomes real. This code explains how people actually find violence and abusive power, for example, erotically stimulating and sexy. "Through such skewed eroticism, people accept in their bodies, as well as in their psyches, that sexism is right and natural, the 'way things are,' and that male gender supremacy feels good."[75]

Except for brief appeals like this one to a critical theory with the power to explain sexual injustice, however, Ellison tends toward generali-

---

73. Ellison, *Erotic Justice,* 1.
74. Gagnon and Simon's classic text is *The Sexual Scene,* John H. Gagnon and William Simon, eds. (Chicago: Aldine Publishing Co., 1970).
75. Ellison, *Erotic Justice,* 51.

ties about the negative influence that social injustices wield upon people's experiences of sexuality. The depth of Ellison's commitment to social construction theory, in other words, is unclear. He never quite says, as other theorists do, that the content of sexuality is created by people. He likely shies away from this assertion because, while recognizing the plasticity of sexuality, he also wants to claim that sexuality is distinctly tied to our capacity for love. Its *telos* is embodied love. He seems to want to say that while people's sexual roles are scripted, human sexuality itself remains unscripted. He relies on the image of pollution: Social injustices like patriarchy and racism have polluted sexuality, which otherwise would be a beautiful thing. Social forces have tainted people's capacity to enjoy life-enhancing, intimate sexuality. The following passage illustrates this mode of argumentation:

> Heterosexism and homophobia *pollute* the channels of sexual intimacy on which people depend for open and trustworthy communication. Patriarchal sex *diminishes* our common well-being as males and females and as heterosexual, homosexual, and bisexual persons. In the midst of this oppressive social structure, we can *easily lose* our *authentic* humanity. We can find ourselves *mistaking* mere body sensations for the delight of sensuous touch born of mutual respect. We may yearn for, but cannot easily establish, life-enhancing connections, person to person.[76]

Like all feminist theologians of the erotic, Ellison invokes here the idea of an authentic, genuine erotic/sexuality that men and women would experience but for the social structures constraining them. In their zeal to reclaim positive meanings of the erotic, they maintain that the erotic is fundamentally good but sometimes becomes tainted. Pollution imagery is Ellison's rhetorical strategy for communicating this concept. Like systematic theologies that employ images of pollution, diminishment, and estrangement to explain humanity's fall into sin and evil, he implicitly suggests a primordial, paradisaical sexual intimacy from which human beings are now estranged and must struggle continually to recapture. He implies that original, unpolluted sexuality is somehow more genuine than what we have in the real world. Does this not contradict, or at least challenge, the idea that sexuality is socially constructed? If sexuality is a product of

---

76. Ellison, *Erotic Justice*, 55 (emphasis added).

society's construction, then this relationship has always existed. While Ellison may want to call egalitarian, respectful, and joyful sexual relationships ideal and even normative, he cannot necessarily call them original.

Along similar lines, Ellison critiques the Christian tradition for its failure to provide a positive sexual ethic. He says that the Church has done little to stop the pollution of sexuality by ignoring (and at times even reinforcing) the equation of domination with sexuality and by keeping silent about the goodness of sexuality. Fear, control, and rigidity have instead characterized Christian discourse about sex. Both the conservative and liberal wings of Christianity, he thinks, are guilty of overemphasizing the danger of sexuality and reinforcing negative attitudes toward the human body. In addition, the church is guilty of acquiescing to the social order that creates sexual injustice. All in all, Christianity has handed down a negative legacy to those who would try to build erotic justice: "Christian tradition, including scripture and church teaching, has had a heavy hand in shaping the prevailing body-denying, sex-negative paradigm of human sexuality."[77]

If progressively minded people who care about justice want to build a more liberating Christian ethic, Ellison proposes a methodological shift. First, he calls for a "clear, definitive, and unapologetic break with the Christian tradition's sex-negativity, oppression of women and gay people, and rigidity about right loving and good sex."[78] Second, he proposes a figurative move toward communities that exist at the margin of society, where an alternative ethic stands a chance of surviving because people at the margins are more open to radical change. Communities on the edges, he suggests, can serve as "training sites" for the struggle to create a sex-positive moral discourse. The details of Ellison's methodology need not concern us here, but that he envisions the task as centrally requiring reimagination is important to note:

> Nothing is more important than our capacity to imagine a radically different world. Such envisioning involves trust. We must trust that we are capable of far more than greed, violence, and sexual irresponsibility. We can imagine, and commit ourselves to, the creation

---

77. Ellison, *Erotic Justice*, 59.
78. Ellison, *Erotic Justice*, 75.

of a radical new world in which all belong and no one's beauty is denied.[79]

Ellison is confident in people's capacity (at least in those who are "progressive") for imagining a decisive and positive alternative to traditional constructions of the erotic:

> We have the capacity to comprehend the power of the erotic in our lives and make good choices about its use. . . . Progressive seekers of justice-love can well imagine living by an ethical eroticism that enjoys life's pleasures and at the same time prods us to pursue a more ethical world.[80]

Ellison's impulse is laudable. The shift he calls for is not irresponsible, and the Christian tradition no doubt awaits decisive change in its sexual ethic. Whether Ellison's methodological shift, however, represents realistic hope for change remains an open question. Radical reimagination of a better world, free from the pernicious influences of social structures, may be needed. But grappling seriously with the reality that the erotic is "grounded" in ever fluctuating social patterns that are often less than ideal might be more helpful in the short run. While human beings may be capable of more than greed, violence, and sexual irresponsibility, some of us will probably always be greedy, violent, and irresponsible with our sexuality. Although the erotic is not by definition a hostile, alien force, neither by definition is the erotic grounded in respect and love. Sometimes the erotic may assume the shape of hostility, sometimes that of love. Moreover, while we are capable of making good choices about its use, our capacity may be limited, and we may simply have to live with the struggle of making better rather than worse choices. Therefore, perhaps our eroticism is not what merits confidence, but the habits of self-care and trust in others that we painstakingly learn and practice over time. In this light, Ellison's project runs the risk of being overly idealistic and even naive.[81]

---

79. Ellison, *Erotic Justice*, 91.

80. Ellison, *Erotic Justice*, 81.

81. I should point out that chapter 5 of Ellison's book avoids this risk. Ellison's analysis of sexual violence in this chapter is critical, careful, and even sobering. Regarding men's potential for reversing their own inculcation in violence, for example, he writes that "pride as well as shame is a valuable moral resource for men, but not all pride is liberating" (111).

Does an identifiable erotic that has escaped captivity by outside influence and that we can tap into to change our world really exist? This question, which we have faced in one way or another in all our feminist theologies of the erotic, arises again in Ellison's work. The question is whether the erotic is basically sound and reliable but has just been taken captive by sexism, heterosexism, and so forth, so that when set free the erotic will be restored to the essential goodness it had "before" captivity; or whether human eroticism has always been and will always be to some extent captured and defined by sin and injustice, so that freedom is not needed so much as continual vigilance. If the erotic is captured by gender injustice and other kinds of injustice, but not finally and irreducibly so (a reasonable compromise), then remedying injustice will remedy the erotic. But progress will be slow and painstaking.

Remedying injustice and the erotic must also be a collective process. Despite his appropriate insistence that the erotic and the political are joined, Ellison still maintains the view that an unspoiled erotic lies trapped within individuals. This view is overly optimistic insofar as Ellison remains too confident that individual human beings have a resource within themselves for finding their own way back to erotic justice. Individuals have, he says, a "place immediately accessible to them — their own body space, as well as their intimate connections with others — within which to mount resistance to injustice and also experiment with freedom."[82]

Ellison misses a factor in the reconstructive task. Resistance is not "immediately accessible" to the oppressed. If the erotic is as deeply constructed as he claims (down to the "somatic" level), then people's body space and their intimate connections with others both will be affected by the various forms of social oppression that need resistance. People cannot find on their own access to a way out. More realistic would be to call for a collective dismantling and rebuilding of erotic experiences, the need for which Ellison seems to recognize at several points but does not connect to his other claims about the erotic. If the "bad news" is social and political, then so must be the "good news." Ellison ultimately contradicts himself because despite starting with claims about the social and political order, he continually returns to the individual's own body space as the site of resistance.

To summarize our discussion of feminist theological discourse about

---

82. Ellison, *Erotic Justice,* 1.

the erotic, we must conclude that certain assumptions hamper its effectiveness in building a sexual ethic. Feminist theologians of the erotic are overly confident that they know the true meaning of erotic experience and that this meaning can be (re)captured by referring to the special female capacities of love, sensuality, relationality, and wisdom. They think that if these capacities are named and lifted up, women (and men) will finally recognize the means to their own freedom — means that, like Dorothy's magic red shoes, they have had all along but failed to employ. The feminist theologians of the erotic contend that erotic oppression works by obscuring people's own innate knowledge of the erotic — that social, political, and religious forces conspire to keep women and men in the dark. Finally, these theologians argue that liberation will come when the real meaning of Eros is pried free and claimed for all the world by people who champion it.

As I show in the next chapter, the general pattern these arguments follow is familiar to people who have tracked feminist theological discourse over the years. Its pitfalls are the same as ones that can be identified within larger debates about appeals to the nature of women and women's experience. Feminist theologies of the erotic are compromised by the same appeals other feminist theologies make to women's experience, that is, to a universal category of experience commonly known by all women. Such appeals served a historical purpose but are now problematic and must be avoided in the search for a workable ethic.

THREE

Considering the Erotic
as Problem

One is *made* a woman.
— Simone de Beauvoir, *The Second Sex*

MANY NONTHEOLOGIANS who write on sexuality today increasingly argue that we are at a crossroads with respect to sexual ethics
and that no obvious or easy direction awaits us. As historian Jeffrey Weeks
states in his widely regarded book, *Sexuality and Its Discontents:*

> We live . . . between worlds, between a world of habits, expectations
> and beliefs that are no longer viable, and a future that has yet to be
> constructed. This gives to sexuality a curiously unsettled and trou-
> bling status: source of pain as much as pleasure, anxiety as much as
> affirmation, identity crisis as much as stability of self.[1]

Theological ethicists need to be at least this honest. Certainly many adolescents today find themselves "between worlds" with respect to sexuality.
As suggested in the introduction, gone are the days when sexual activity
automatically signaled that two people were in love and would eventually
marry (or were already married). People simply no longer widely concur
that marriage is or should be the *telos* of adolescent sexuality. While more
people agree that adolescents should wait until they are "in love," neither
is this expectation unanimous. Agreement on such expectations, as Weeks
puts it, is less and less viable. At the same time, no consensus about the
moral meaning and purpose of sexuality has yet emerged for adolescents
to grasp.

Yet feminist theologies of the erotic all begin with the same basic conviction: A distorted or thwarted Eros lies at the heart of most human

---

1. Jeffrey Weeks, *Sexuality and Its Discontents* (London: Routledge & Kegan Paul, 1985), 3.

60

misery (in sexuality and beyond). Their primary remedy is to identify a "true" Eros that has been taken captive inside people but which, were it only released, would help people see the light and turn their misery into happiness. In other words, according to feminist theologies of the erotic, the problem is that forces like sexism, heterosexism, and body hatred render impossible people knowing what authentic erotic experiences are like. Such forces pervert the real meaning of Eros, which is good, and twist it into something false, which is bad. Misconception takes Eros captive. Real Eros is about intimacy and mutuality and love, but people are misled into believing otherwise and are therefore temporarily rendered incapable of leading fulfilling, wholesome sex lives. Thus, feminist theologians of the erotic see their imperative to be breaking the shackles of tradition that hold Eros captive. They argue for a sanctification and blessing of Eros, and they encourage its expression. Once people are morally legitimated as sexual and erotic beings, they argue, they will be freed from the fear and repression of their passions and will be able to affirm and even celebrate their eroticism.

What could be wrong with doing sexual ethics this way? Initially finding fault with feminist theologies of the erotic is difficult, for their approach sounds liberating — indeed, even new and refreshing — and especially appropriate to adolescents' stirrings for freedom and fulfillment. But problems exist, not least of which are its implications for an ethic for adolescent sexuality. Let me outline five problems and suggest some lines of thinking that would begin to correct them, drawn primarily from sources outside theology.

Challenges to Feminist Theologies of the Erotic

First, as appealing as it may be, the positive sanctioning of Eros risks overgeneralization and naiveté. Feminist theologians of the erotic imply that erotic passion should be liberated because it is always good — at least so long as its expression is not abusive. But the caveat is inadequate. Even after we rule out clearly abusive desires (such as a desire to rape or a desire for sex with children), whether all sexual passion should be automatically sanctioned as unequivocally good remains questionable. Less blatantly harmful desires lodge in the psyche and also cause misery in time. For example, a yearning to be swept away as in the fairy tales; a predilection for quick, impersonal sex; a craving to be constantly seduced;

an attraction to domineering sexual partners — modes of desire that are often particularly compelling to adolescents — are all desires whose indulgence might well be inadvisable. Simply put, not all kinds of sexual desiring are good for us, but desiring that might in the end be bad cannot be addressed if it is not even recognized. Moreover, in some people, Eros is so muted that "repression" seems an insufficient explanation for the alienation they experience in their sexual lives, and the sanctioning of passion is an insufficient remedy. Therefore, instead of assuming that the erotic is always good, we might rather question such a serious disconnection from something that is supposedly "natural," good, and accessible to every person *qua* human person.

Focusing on liberation from suppression or repression of erotic passion, as feminist theologians do, suggests that persons know what they desire but feel inhibited or restrained in expressing it. Once the barriers of inhibition are lifted, so the logic goes, passion flowers. But is this line of thinking adequate? The individual does have significant power to change her conception and experience of the erotic if the primary problem is repression and the primary remedy individual liberation. But as Michel Foucault persuasively argues, a "repressive hypothesis" needs to be supplanted or at least supplemented by an examination of the reasons that some people have the power to define and repress other people's sexuality at all.[2]

Therefore, in addition to a tendency toward naiveté, a second problem with feminist theologies of the erotic is their tendency to overlook the necessary analyses of power relations and gender built into the erotic itself. These theologies are likely to miss the collective, rather than purely individual, wielding of power that shapes and transforms sexuality, without an appreciation of which sexual passion cannot fully be understood. Most of the theologians reviewed here appreciate the ways societal forces (like sexism and homophobia) have hurt and confused people erotically; they all decry discrimination, abuse, and oppression of all kinds. But if the proposed remedy to these sorts of injustices is for individuals to access their erotic power, as feminist theologians of the erotic suggest, then individuals thus "liberated" will only be liberated to a world in which these forces still reign, and this advance will not be significant.

The problem is that social and cultural conditions continually interact

---

2. Michel Foucault, *The History of Sexuality,* vol. 1 (New York: Random House, 1978), part 2.

with eroticism, producing what people find erotic. This activity goes on all the time, generating what people understand the very meaning of the erotic to be at any given time. The erotic inclinations and desires that feminist theologians urge us to access are gendered — and racialized and so forth — from the start. (We see this in chapter 5, where I trace back to early childhood girls' desire for romance and their inclination to disavow themselves.) Therefore, despite their indisputable concern for women, feminist theologians of the erotic miss something crucial when they fail to attend to the interplay of gender and power and the systematic influence these forces have on sexuality. Exerting more individual willpower will never change the content of eroticism radically enough.

A third, related shortcoming in feminist theologies of the erotic lies with the tendency to essentialize. They run the risk of assuming an invariable core or kernel within human sexuality (or human passion more generally) that is "the erotic." But if one posits an original, authentic Eros that needs to be unearthed and emancipated, one is assuming that an erotic exists in some primordial realm "before" captivity, as suggested in the preceding chapter, implying that all persons share an identifiable erotic in basically the same form. In other words, a shared essence to the erotic can be identified and known apart from concrete historical instances of it. Whatever one thinks of essentialism in general, it raises special difficulties in the sexual sphere and should be avoided.

Today, both ordinary wisdom and theory problematize the claim that all people's sexual experiences share some common core. Many secular feminist theorists, in particular, increasingly doubt that sexual experience, or any gendered experience for that matter, has any identifiable essence. They emphasize instead the plasticity and historical specificity of human experience. In other words, the meanings of sexuality and Eros are socially constructed, not timelessly given (as Ellison acknowledges). They are not merely elements of human nature affected by social conditions; rather, the very forms we employ to interpret and speak about, and therefore shape, our sexuality are constructed out of the social fabric we wear.

These three problems — the lurking naiveté of feminist theologies of the erotic, their blind spot with regard to the way power works upon sexuality, and their tendency toward a strong essentialism — suggest the need for an ethic informed by a different sort of theory about sexuality. One alternative might evolve from Foucault and others who affirm that Eros is socially produced or constructed. What does it mean to talk about the "construction" of the erotic? Foucault argues that sexual desire is a site of power relations between people. Power is not alien to sex, he says, controlling or repressing it from some external vantage point, as commonly thought, but rather sex is a medium through which power is created and exchanged. Hence, sexual desires are configured and produced differently according to changes in the power relations that flow between and among people. Foucault did not have in mind the wielding of power only by large institutions or even social systems like the church, the capitalist state, or the family. He argues that power is diffuse, present in and reproduced by all everyday discourse about sex. Indeed, the proliferation of anxious talk about and preoccupation with sex has more to do with its construction in our collective understanding than does anything else, according to Foucault.

Foucaultian presuppositions regarding a theory of sexuality have significant implications for a critique of feminist theologies of the erotic. Such presuppositions contrast sharply with the notion of an eternal, changeless essence to Eros. They raise questions about whether the erotic can even be known and talked about apart from actual historical constructions of it. A feminist theorist who shares many of Foucault's convictions about the socially produced nature of sexuality, Catharine MacKinnon, argues that women cannot know really enjoyable sex because sex as they know and experience it is entirely a product of patriarchal culture. MacKinnon "defines" sexuality as follows:

> Sexuality, in its feminist light, is not a discrete sphere of interaction or feeling or sensation or behavior in which preexisting social divisions may or not be played out. It is a pervasive dimension of social life, one that permeates the whole, a dimension along which gender occurs and through which gender is socially constituted. . . . So many distinct features of women's status as second class — the restriction and constraint and contortion, the servility and the display, the self-mutilation and requisite presentation of self as a beautiful thing, the enforced passivity, the humiliation — are made into the content of sex for women.[3]

This definition connects sexuality to women's second-class status and makes it a product of, rather than producer of, social interchange between

---

3. Catharine MacKinnon, *Toward a Feminist Theory of the State* (Cambridge, Mass.: Harvard University Press, 1989), 130.

women and men. Such a perspective departs radically from feminist theologies of the erotic; what we have now is Eros continually constituted out of the seemingly timeless divisions of gender.

A social constructionist theory of sexuality also challenges the view that repression is the main problem in people's erotic lives. Such a view assumes an Eros pried free from power dynamics, but according to Foucault's theory, no such thing can exist. Finally, a theory that accepts the social construction of Eros is less hopeful about reaching a point in time when destructive Eros will be overthrown and replaced by authentic, good Eros. This theory suggests a more sober approach to ethics. At the same time, such an approach may be more sanguine about interim possibilities for erotic pleasure and joy because the enjoyment of sex is not dependent upon some final overthrow of oppressive institutions.[4]

To accept a social constructionist theory of the erotic is not to say that people never experience the erotic in a way that is their own. To claim that desires are "socially constructed" or produced does not mean that they are fabricated, unreal, or not truly the desires of particular desiring subjects. Neither does this claim require that we deny the validity of people who say that their desires are authentic to them. Desires bear the stamp of individual people and often feel "given" in the sense of being spontaneous. We all surely feel our feelings immediately, acutely, and spontaneously. Rather, what social construction means is that we can never be sure that the *meaning* we assign to our desires is entirely of our own making. Desires never come to us already fully vested with meaning; to the contrary, their meaning develops and changes as it is employed over time and from context to context and culture to culture. As Mary McClintock Fulkerson argues in defense of feminist arguments about the social construction of the body: "When we treat bodies as constructed, it is not their existence that we call into question, but the fixed character of their meaning."[5] At one level, feminist theologians of the erotic are correct to say that individuals experience the erotic as a blessed gift, a precious part of God's good creation. Individuals' experiences of yearning, passion, and pleasure are genuine and should be appreciated as such. But what cannot be so eas-

---

4. This point may be one on which Catharine MacKinnon differs from Foucault. MacKinnon's logic allows room for imagining a future realm in which patriarchy will be overthrown, but renders more pessimistic our view of present realities.

5. Mary McClintock Fulkerson, *Changing the Subject: Women's Discourses and Feminist Theology* (Minneapolis: Fortress Press, 1994), 88.

ily affirmed is the meaning of those yearnings and pleasures — why they develop, what they stand for, and whether they are unambiguously praise-worthy. Feminist theologians of the erotic are therefore mistaken to think that its meaning is readily accessible, transparent, and always liberatory.

Additional Concerns with Feminist Theologies of the Erotic

Letting go of the assumption that the meanings of sexual experience are always clear and liberatory would alleviate a fourth problem we can identify in feminist theologies of the erotic, which is a tendency toward overconfident libertarian thinking. These theologians assume not only that women's experience of the erotic is transparent but that the more delving into it the better. Combining this approach with a desire to affirm the naturalness and guiltlessness of women's experience of the erotic, they effectively communicate a "Go for it!" message. As we have seen, they encourage women actively to unearth their repressed erotic desires and to treasure whatever they discover. Such a message could be construed as an invitation to undisciplined revelry in any and all erotic expressions, thus valuing the freedom of Eros over the quality of Eros.

This message assumes, however, that women's immediate interpretation of their experience is sufficient and trustworthy, needing no other sources for interpretation, as if women can know what their feelings mean if they just feel them intensely enough. "Deep down," the assumption goes, women really know what they want and have only to rid themselves of whatever has hindered them from acknowledging and voicing their de-sires. Once they purge their thinking of bad ideology, they will have no more problems. Patriarchy in this view is like clothing one can remove, rather than like a coiled knot of oppressions that requires systematic dis-entangling.[6] As I will show later in this book, for example, many young women have been told that nothing shameful about their bodies or their desires exists, and they genuinely believe this statement at some level. In other words, they are not simply mired in false ideology. Yet they are still painfully aware that they cannot articulate what they want (or do not

---

6. See Sandra Bartky's "Feminine Masochism and the Politics of Personal Transformation," in *Philosophy of Sex: Contemporary Readings,* 2d ed., ed. Alan Soble (Savage, Md.: Rowman and Littlefield, 1991), 233. Bartky is critical of feminists who think that dismantling "the ideological apparatus of patriarchal society" suffices to recondition desire (233).

want) sexually. They know, as some psychologists put it, about their own "not knowing." Some girls even suspect that their confusion is tied to their being female. They cannot just apply more courage and confidence to their erotic desiring. In short, they are both more astute and more troubled than feminist theologies of the erotic are able to appreciate. Again, the conclusion should not be that girls and women never experience a simple, immediate, "gut" sense of desire that they can name and trust. To express skepticism about the reliability of experience is not to deny the existence of an experiencing subject who can claim her own thoughts and feelings, but to deny the ease of thinking one's way out of confusing experiences.

Feminist theologians' overconfident, libertarian attitude could be called "sex-positivity," contrasting them with the sex-negative thinkers they criticize. Sex-positive thinkers believe that all sexual expression should be presumed morally good, unless proven otherwise, and that people should therefore be free to choose whatever sexual expression they want.[7] But a sex-positive theology can become, when taken to an extreme, so optimistic that it eschews the need for moral boundaries. Philosopher Sandra Bartky identifies a version of sex-positivity she calls "sexual voluntarism," which is the presumption that individual women can will their own sexual freedom. Bartky critiques sexual voluntarism on two grounds. Not only does it ignore the depth of the damage that oppression can cause, she says, but it also ironically casts women in a solo role, each woman individually lifting her own oppression.

> "Any woman can" — such is the motto of voluntarism. Armed with an adequate feminist critique of sexuality and sufficient will power, any woman should be able to alter the pattern of her own desires . . . those who claim that any woman can reprogram her consciousness if only she is sufficiently determined hold a shallow view of the nature of patriarchal oppression. Anything done can be undone, it is implied, nothing has been permanently damaged, nothing irretrievably lost.[8]

While Bartky was responding to other philosophers, her criticisms apply to feminist theologians of the erotic as well. Because of their optimism about

---

7. Interestingly enough, in moral discourse "sex-positive" is a term used by its opponents and proponents alike. Some ethicists like Ellison, for example, take pride in being sex-positive. But one can also find the term being used disparagingly.

8. Bartky, "Feminine Masochism and the Politics of Personal Transformation," 234.

the erotic, they come dangerously close to substituting voluntarism for
the sober critical analysis that today's sexual ethics requires. They assume
that a pure, untroubled experience of the erotic is available immediately
to every woman given enough "deprogramming." But voluntarism alone
will not succeed in reconciling us with the erotic.

A fifth and final problem within feminist theologies of the erotic lies
in the norms they propose for sexual life. As we have seen, feminist theologians of the erotic put great stress on relationality in their discourse
about the erotic as one of the primary norms they promote for sexual and
other relationships. They also believe that the erotic by itself naturally in-
vites relationships of greater relationality. I have already pointed out some
of the dangers of this type of discourse, such as its danger for girls and
women who tend more than boys and men to overinvest in relationship —
so keenly sometimes that they run the risk of subsuming their particular
needs and desires under the other's. As we see in the next chapter, the
tendency of adolescent girls to orient themselves toward relationship at
times imperils their integrity and sense of self. In such cases, relationality
becomes the very trait of the female erotic to critique, not the trait to
celebrate. Yet feminist theologies of the erotic often ironically glorify the
very things that need critical scrutiny. Therefore, structuring any ethic,
but especially a sexual ethic, so solidly around the values of relationality
proves redundant for many women and girls. In more theoretical terms,
autonomy must balance relationality. To borrow an argument of feminist
theorist Seyla Benhabib:

> When the story of a life can only be told from the standpoint of
> the individual, then such a self is a narcissist and a loner who may
> have attained autonomy without solidarity. When the story of a life
> can only be told from the standpoint of the others, then the self
> is a victim and sufferer who has lost control over her existence. A
> coherent sense of self is attained with the successful integration of
> solidarity and autonomy.[9]

To build a more adequate sexual ethic, we need to identify a different norm. Whatever we call it — be it "relationality" or "mutuality" or
"trust" — the norm must be a quality of *relationship*, not a personality

---

9. Seyla Benhabib, "The Debate Over Women and Moral Theory Revisited," in *Situating
the Self: Gender, Community and Postmodernism in Contemporary Ethics* (New York: Routledge,
1992), 198.

profile or a virtue we praise in individuals. We do not need to stop talking about these norms, but we need to be clear that they are not reducible to attending ever more closely to the other and certainly should not mean a blurring beyond recognition of the boundaries between other and self.

Given these five problems, we can question the wisdom of a continuing move to sexual ethics in the direction proposed by feminist theologians of the erotic. In their overconfidence, they neglect important concerns that still trouble many other theorists, not to mention many individuals who struggle to live decent sexual lives. Indeed, in the introduction to *Touching Our Strength,* Heyward admits that her book is written for a specific audience:

> I am attempting to give voice to an embodied — sensual — relational movement among women and men who experience our sexualities as a liberating resource and who, at least in part through this experience, have been strengthened in the struggle for justice for all.[10]

In contrast, ethicists need to bear in mind people who in this movement have been left behind. Many girls and women do not experience their sexualities as liberating resources and rarely, if ever, draw upon their sexual experience as a resource in their pursuit of justice. Many have not yet discovered the erotic as a source of power in their sexual relationships, let alone in their "language and history and work," as Lorde claimed. Many find the sexual and erotic aspects of their lives still greatly diminished in quality or even missing entirely and think erotic passion simply connotes being a slut — or having a boyfriend. They judge erotic experiences to be *sometimes* joyously significant, but just as often banal. For many individuals, the erotic is a long way from opening them to multiple dimensions of joy, as Lorde put it in 1978.

The vision that Lorde and Heyward and others hold out has undeniable value, but all of us cannot seem to get there.[11] Feminist theologians of the erotic have paved the way to a much more liberating discussion about sexuality than was previously possible. Traditional approaches to sexual ethics that emphasized control and rigidity were admittedly distasteful, hurtful, and inadequate. But will the approach of liberating the erotic,

---

10. Heyward, *Touching Our Strength,* 3.

11. For framing the problem this way, I am indebted to one of my students at Oberlin College, Polly Dondy-Kaplan, in conversation December 1996. I am grateful to all the students in my course on sexual ethics who helped me think through Lorde's essay.

on the other hand, suffice? As important as aspiring to erotic liberation
is, affirmation of the erotic's positive meanings does not alone create a
sexual ethic that can withstand the complexities of everyone's experiences.
Somehow the idea has not borne fruit that the celebration of Eros alone
will create a liberatory new paradigm for sexual attitudes and behavior, at
least according to many young women.

Feminist Theologies of the Erotic in Context

Because the erotic is more a problem that still needs reckoning with than
it is a solution to a problem, an ethic for adolescent sexuality will have
serious flaws if it is grounded in the kind of theology I am calling feminist theology of the erotic. To understand better the shortcomings in this
kind of theological thinking, we might ask what generates them in the
first place. In other words, what theological assumptions — particularly
about women and the nature of their experiences — lead these feminists
to place such faith in the erotic and count on it to be so liberating? If
we can uncover the logic of their confident discourse, we can mount a
stronger critique. Illumination of feminist theologies of the erotic is aided
if we place them within the historical context of the development of feminist theology. Feminist theological discourse about the erotic not only
responds to traditional (nonfeminist) theology but also to earlier feminist
work. This discourse can furthermore be contrasted with still newer feminist theologies. In other words, to discern more clearly alternative ways
of doing sexual ethics, placing feminist theologians of the erotic on the
feminist map can help. What follows in this section, therefore, is a brief
historical sketch of types of feminist theology and an argument that feminist theologies of the erotic fall within what can be called "experiential
feminism."

Experiential feminism is the belief that a core of human experiences
called "women's experience" exists which serves to test the normative value
of theological and ethical claims about God's purpose for human life. As
Sheila Greeve Davaney argues, many feminists in the "first wave" of feminist theology shared certain assumptions (without necessarily realizing it)
about women's experience, especially in its relation to divine purpose. She
identifies four main ideas that she calls "working assumptions" of early
feminist theology. They are (a) that women's experience has a common
core; (b) that women's experience is a normative site against which theo-

logical claims can be tested; (c) that the Christian theological tradition, too, has a common core that can be said to function in a similar way; and d) that a correspondence exists between feminist norms and claims about the divine.[12] I submit that feminist theologies of the erotic continue to do theology according to these assumptions, which in part explains the problems cited in the first section of this chapter.

As Davaney points out, the logic of these four assumptions often went unarticulated within early feminist theologies precisely because they were assumptions. Convictions about the uniqueness and value of women and women's experience were so foundational to early feminist theology that they constituted what it meant to do "feminist" theology at all. Only now that claims about women's commonality and the uniqueness of their experience receive direct challenge within feminist thought itself do they become more visible — and, to many, more dubious. Davaney's list of assumptions is helpful because these exact assumptions are coming under fire within feminist theology today; in fact, debate about them occupies a central place within current feminist theological work. Many theologians find these assumptions, to use Davaney's term, too "felicitous" — that is, suspiciously convenient and naive — and lacking theological and philosophical merit. However, other theologians and ethics still subscribe to and actively defend these convictions about women and experience. In other words, although Davaney identifies this set of ideas as belonging to an earlier era, they still hold sway.

The reason they still hold sway is that many feminists recognize that to assume their utter opposite would be unwise and even dangerous for feminism. To assume that women's experiences have nothing at all in common, that there is no normative wisdom to be gained from examining women's experiences, and that the divine is to be understood completely apart from women's experiences, would be to void the categories of "women" and "experience" (and possibly "divine") and to invite nihilism and relativism. Therefore, while strong versions of these claims are increasingly rejected, weaker versions find more acceptance, especially among ethicists, who harbor particular worries about moral nihilism and relativism.

With respect to feminist theologies of the erotic, assumptions a, b, and d are particularly relevant. The questions become: Do women's erotic ex-

---

12. Sheila Greeve Davaney, "Continuing the Story but Departing the Text," in *Horizons in Feminist Theology: Identity, Tradition and Norms,* ed. Rebecca Chopp and Sheila Greeve Davaney (Minneapolis: Fortress Press, 1997), 198–214.

periences share a common core? Does the female erotic carry normative value? Does the female erotic reflect the divine better than the male erotic? A skeptic such as myself will resist answering these questions in the affirmative. And yet I, too, recognize the danger of simply dismissing them. Without recognizing the sacredness of female experience, one limits the divine. Without insisting that girls' and women's voices receive attention — even special attention — within theology, one runs the risk of returning to an era when theological conclusions were drawn exclusively from male experience. And without identifying some commonality among girls' and women's experiences, one cannot offer any moral norms to help.

A Common Women's Experience?

Experiential feminism — again, in its theological form, the belief that a core of human experiences called "women's experience" serves as a plumb line of theology and ethics — arose in response to an even earlier form of feminism, namely, liberal feminism. Liberal feminism was itself a response — to (androcentric) liberal theology and theory. Liberal feminists modified the basic tenets of liberalism, such as the primacy of reason and the importance of individualism to human experience, to include women. They shared with classic liberals a belief in a thing called "human experience" that could be abstracted from everyone's various individual experiences across time and place. What liberal feminists did, however, was to expose the androcentrism of "human experience." They showed how what had been taken to be "human" experience had all along really just been men's experience. In other words, using various strategies, they demonstrated that the experiencing "self" of classic liberal theory was gendered; it was really a male self, not representing women's experiences of selfhood. To correct this stance, they sought to incorporate women and women's experience into liberal theory. The individualistic, reasoning self, they argued, could be male or female. Differences do not matter. As humans, women experience the same things men do. Liberation as a woman comes in being visible and rightfully acknowledged alongside a man.

The feminists I am calling experiential feminists react to liberal feminism by challenging the assumption that women experience the same things men do. Differences do matter, they contend. They find the liberal feminist assumptions of gender parity and similarity to be false and argue instead that women share a common lot that is importantly different from that of men. As the author of one of the first feminist theological texts put it: "It is my contention that there are significant differences between masculine and feminine experience and that feminine experience reveals in a more emphatic fashion certain aspects of the human situation which are present but less obvious in the experience of men."[13] Some experiential feminist theologians locate the basis of women's common experience in biology, others in the dynamics of oppression. In other words, some experiential feminists argue that women's experiences are similar because women share a common nature that is grounded in female embodiment. Others argue that all women share a bond by virtue of being oppressed by patriarchy, which means, both literally and figuratively, the "rule of the fathers." Patriarchal rule, they say, is present and experienced in every dimension of women's lives, including economic, political, and sexual. Liberation for women will arrive "after the patriarchy," that is, when patriarchy is removed.

In this theological framework, experiences of daily life — such as experiences of eroticism — become especially important as both vehicles for and proof of liberation. If one believes that women are *not* "just the same" as men, but their experience is uniquely female, then any evidence of uniquely female experience tends to prove one's point. Stated another way, if one's argument is that experience sets women apart from men (in both negative and positive ways), one cannot help but look hard for commonality within women's diverse experiences. This commonality then serves to form the substance of one's normative claims. As Ada María Isasi-Díaz says:

> Women's experiences are the locus and source of women's liberation theologies. Intrinsic to these theologies is a repudiation of universalist and transhistorical reason, hitherto elaborated and maintained as revelatory and normative by males and patriarchal structures. Instead, the daily experiences of women struggling for liberation have become the core of women's liberation theologies' critical norms.[14]

One example of feminist theologians' of the erotic repudiating liberal reasoning about sexuality is the observation, cited in the previous chapter, that unlike many men, women infrequently become carried away by over-

---

13. Valerie Saiving Goldstein, "The Human Situation: A Feminine View," *Journal of Religion* 40 (1960). If female experience only shows more clearly "the human situation," however, this thinking would be classically liberal.

14. Ada María Isasi-Díaz, "Experiences," *Dictionary of Feminist Theologies,* ed. Letty M. Russell and J. Shannon Clarkson (Louisville, Ky.: Westminster/John Knox Press, 1996), 95.

whelming, unrestrained sexual desire. The long-held philosophical and theological assumption that sexual desire is irresistible turned out to be based on many *men's* difficulty resisting it — an experience women do not generally share. If women's experience resisting sexual desire were taken to be the norm, theologians might form a very different view of Eros.

Moreover, evidence of a unique and flourishing "female experience" can function to show the extent to which women have already been freed, if only because they can name their own experiences *as women*. (Simply by identifying their different history of sexual desiring, to continue the example, women come to know themselves as uniquely female and gain the confidence to reject androcentric assumptions about sexuality.) Identifying common female experience becomes the key to liberation, because the experience both justifies the need for liberation and creates solidarity so that liberation will eventually result.[15] The lifting up and naming of experience, which is the basis for the struggle against oppression, itself carries moral meaning and significance to experiential feminists. Simply the fact of claiming an experience to be women's experience carries great power for them.[16] Even if women's commonality lies in their oppression by men, by naming it one hints at a female experience that exists behind the layers of that oppression and looks eschatologically toward a time when female experience will "rule," figuratively if not literally. Hope thus lies in the identification and expression of that which is known through distinctly female experience.

Another example of the repudiation of liberal thinking can be found in Rita Nakashima Brock's claim that women have developed a special form of cognition called "knowing by heart." She explicitly contrasts knowing by heart with androcentric reasoning; the latter is detached and objective

---

15. Feminist consciousness-raising groups of the 1960s and '70s held this logic, which some feminists have recently called for again. See, for example, bell hooks, "Sisterhood: Solidarity between Women" in *Feminist Theory: From Margin to Center* (Boston: South End Press, 1984). It is important to note that hooks's concept of solidarity calls for women working together across lines of race and class, a feature often missing in the early consciousness-raising groups.

16. The power of naming is especially vivid in the earliest feminist theological texts, whose primary task was to clear up longstanding misconceptions about women. In them one can hear an insistent voice claiming that the real meaning of women's experience is not necessarily what it has always been thought to be. For example, Judith Plaskow began her book, *Sex, Sin and Grace* by contrasting mythologies *about* women (especially Freudian and Jungian theories about women's passivity) with stories *by* women. "What I call 'women's situation' or 'women's experience' has two interrelated aspects: what has been said about women, mostly by men, and the ways in which women have experienced themselves." *Sex, Sin and Grace: Women's Experience and the Theologies of Reinhold Niebuhr and Paul Tillich* (Washington, D.C.: University Press of America, 1980), 9.

rather than passionate and subjective. Women have had special opportunities to practice knowing by heart, Brock claims, and have consequently nurtured it into a powerful, passionate form of wisdom that is uniquely feminine. The point is that Brock's identification and celebration of this type of wisdom is a direct response to liberal theory about how people know what they know.

We can see why feminist theologians of the erotic consider powerful the very naming and claiming of female erotic experience. Naming and claiming justify what androcentric theology has hitherto dismissed — women's sexuality and passion — and the ideas that follow when these forces become the focus. The mere fact of recognizing that women experience eroticism in a different way from men challenges previous assumptions and shifts emphases within theology and ethics.

From embracing the importance of naming and claiming women's experience to making it uniform, however, is a short step. The temptation, and the danger, of this type of feminist thought is to gloss over differences in women's experiences to find a common essence that is distinctly female. Therefore, one of the main criticisms leveled against experiential feminists, whether of the biologist or oppressionist sort, is, to put it crudely, that they merely replace "masculine" with "feminine." Linell Elizabeth Cady, who uses the term "essentialist feminism" for what I am calling experiential feminism, writes:

> Explicitly rejecting the veil of neutrality that surrounds the liberal construal of the subject, essentialist feminism tags it as "male" and seeks to articulate its "female" counterpart. Significant effort has been directed to charting, for example, a distinctively female moral development or women's ways of knowing. This work clearly contributes to combating the fictitious neutrality in the myth of liberalism which helps to secure its hegemony. However, it does so by duplicating some of the moves by which liberalism achieves its supposed unity and universality. The female subject purportedly shares a common identity with other women and a common experience of oppression. Built into essentialist feminism is the propensity to secure unity through abstract homogeneity, a procedure that reflects the same ahistorical tendencies of the alternative it rejects.[17]

---

17. Linell Elizabeth Cady, "Identity, Feminist Theory, and Theology" in *Horizons,* ed. Chopp and Davaney, "Continuing the Story but Departing the Text," 21.

One cannot discount the contribution that feminist theologians of the erotic have made to theological thinking about women and sexuality. They have shown that women and men are not the same in their ways of erotic loving. They have also effectively demonstrated the many ways women are oppressed erotically. We have reaped value, in other words, from their arguments, indeed, even from their generalizations, about women and the erotic. And yet, one can also see how tempting it can be to feminist theologians of the erotic to disregard important differences among women and to assume commonality just when questioning it might be more important. One can additionally see how easy it would be to become uncritical of women's experience, or, to put it differently, how difficult it might be to critique the sexual and erotic experiences of women. Confidence in the existence of a "female erotic" is essential to a liberationist message, in the same way that evidence of common female experience motivates experiential feminism. Different feminist theologians of the erotic subscribe to different theories for what generates the "common core" of women's experiences of sex and Eros. Some assume it to be primarily sociocultural (Ellison), others, psychological (Brock). But all have in some way utilized the idea of a common core to make their liberationist claims. Set against the backdrop of liberal feminism, we can better understand why feminist theologians of the erotic contend that the female erotic has the power to liberate women.

Women's Experience as Normative?

Davaney's second point is that beyond assuming a common core at the heart of women's experience, many of the early feminist theologians assumed that core itself to carry normative weight — as she puts it, they assumed experience to be a "site" against which theological and ethical claims could be tested. If a theory or doctrine did not resonate with everyday, lived experience, then that theory or doctrine needed modification or replacement. Another way of putting this idea is to say that early feminist theologians made experience authoritative. The logic went something like this: "If so many women experience x, that must prove some profound truth." Sometimes that logic became: "If so many women experience x, then any ideology that calls x wrong must itself be wrong."

Much discussion takes place in feminist theological ethics about the relationship of experience to theological and ethical claims. For example, in the normative sphere, feminist ethicists have raised such questions as the following: Given the terrible experience of battered wives, must the biblical laws against divorce always be obeyed?[18] Can something like homoerotic love be morally unacceptable that is experienced, by lesbians, as so good?[19] In the sphere of methodological ethics, feminists ask about the relative authorities of text, tradition, and testimony.[20] They offer arguments for letting women's experience serve as a judge of, or at least boundary around, interpretations of scripture and tradition that have ethical import for women's lives.

Feminist theologians of the erotic continue this same line of thinking by asking: Can Eros really be so dangerous if it feels so right? They argue that moral wisdom flows from the experience of erotic passion, and that this wisdom ought to carry some weight against traditional ethical logic that calls Eros dangerous and discourages its expression. Feminist theologies of the erotic are not only saying that women have tapped into a wellspring of vitality and power that should receive notice, but also that erotic vitality and power should serve as a measure against which any potentially sexist/heterosexist/racist content within theology is tested.

We can raise three kinds of concerns about the assumption that women's experience serves as a normative site in doing theological ethics. One concern is that in giving away too much moral authority to experience, scripture and tradition are divested of it, as though experience were given a trump card in establishing the moral norms for the community. This possibility bothers some who not only worry that experience may be fickle and flimsy but who also object to a theological ethics that appears ungrounded in the historical texts and teachings of the Christian faith.[21]

A second concern, felt keenly today within the feminist theological community, is whether in deciding to value experience as a normative site, one does not have to decide *whose* experience to value. Moral norms are presumed to be valid for the whole community, but does not the privileg-

---

18. See, for example, Susan Brooks Thistlethwaite, "Every Two Minutes: Battered Women and Feminist Interpretation," in *Weaving the Visions: New Patterns in Feminist Spirituality,* ed. Judith Plaskow and Carol P. Christ (San Francisco: HarperSanFrancisco, 1989).

19. See Gilson, *Eros Breaking Free;* Heyward's other books, including *Staying Power: Reflections on Gender, Justice, and Compassion* (Cleveland: Pilgrim Press, 1995); and Alison R. Webster, *Found Wanting: Women, Christianity, and Sexuality* (London: Cassell, 1995).

20. See, for example, "Feminist Consciousness and the Interpretation of Scripture," in *Feminist Interpretation of the Bible,* ed. Letty M. Russell (Philadelphia: Westminster Press, 1985).

21. See, for example, David Hollenbach, "Tradition, History, and Truth in Theological Ethics," 60–75, and Gene Outka, "The Particularist Turn in Theological and Philosophical Ethics," 93–118, in *Christian Ethics: Problems and Prospects,* ed. Lisa Sowle Cahill and James Childress (Cleveland: Pilgrim Press, 1996).

ing of experience necessarily mean privileging some people's experience over others'? (A similar question, called the question of canon, has been raised of scriptures and teachings. Thus, the issue of concern might be called the canonizing of experience.)

A third concern, perhaps most relevant to our project, is whether people's experiences can simply be taken at face value. Does "experience" interpret itself so easily that it can stand as a stable, comprehensible "site" against which norms for something like sexual behavior can be tested? Is the meaning of women's experience so apparent that it can be located, let alone granted normative status? Does one not run the risk of assuming "experience" comes vested with meaning, needing no further examination or interpretation? These questions cause the second assumption of experiential feminism to erode. The complexity and opacity of most human experiences rich enough to generate moral wisdom prevent them from being directly revelatory.

Feminist theologies of the erotic are susceptible to these concerns and criticisms because they, too, assume experience to be a normative site. Their logic goes like this: Women are oppressed by virtue of their eroticism and are denied equal access to the fullness of life that privileged heterosexual men enjoy. The cause of their oppression is a patriarchal society and religion that perpetuate sexism, heterosexism, racism, and classism, and distort and destroy women's experience of the erotic. But women's real experience of the erotic, the one they would enjoy were it not for their oppression, is the truth and is liberating. Some women are lucky enough to have had this real experience and to have discovered the truth about Eros. They should lead the way in advocating erotic liberation for all. Once liberated to the real meaning of the erotic, all women will experience its full power and glory.

If we remind ourselves that the purpose of asserting the "real truth" about women's erotic is to counter sexist, androcentric misconceptions, we can be sympathetic to what feminist theologians of the erotic are doing. Their goal is to transform traditional thinking about the erotic by affirming a different vision, based upon previously ignored accounts of experience. But their logic positions them in a perpetual negative dialectic, always testing against women's experience what the tradition has done to Eros — and usually saying no to tradition. No wonder feminist theologians refer so often to Audre Lorde's cry of "Yes!" "Yes" is the answer to the tradition's "No"; one says "Yes" to freedom and liberation to escape the negativity of distortion and destruction. Indeed, Ellison explicitly describes his project as a "break" from tradition: "In order to craft [a liberating Christian sexual ethic], we must make a clear, definitive, and unapologetic break with the Christian tradition's sex-negativity, oppression of women and gay people, and rigidity about right loving and good sex."[22]

Admittedly, the strategy of feminist theologians of the erotic succeeds in exposing all the damage, deformation, and distortion that society and religion inflict upon women's lives. They have made us aware of the crazy ways women's sexuality has been portrayed and of all the oppressing conditions that stifle that sexuality. The problem with assuming this kind of dialectical stance vis-à-vis tradition, however, is the risk of ignoring the power of "*wrong* loving and *bad* sex." Women's pain may be so soundly rejected that it is, in effect, denied any reality or power. Yet women's experience is still genuinely "distorted," and the problem is that so-called distortions are produced and reproduced so often and so thoroughly in women's lives that they begin to seem like more than distortions. What feminist theologians of the erotic call a falsity feels real and compelling to many girls and women.

We are thus led to wonder: Why are not all women able to have the "real" erotic experiences feminist theologians of the erotic talk about? Why do problems with Eros linger so long in many women's lives if the issue is simply a matter of saying "No" to traditional ideologies about the erotic? Given that sexual and erotic liberation is now within so many women's grasp, do women who remain oppressed have themselves to blame? Does their difficulty stem from failing to embrace the "Yes!"? From letting themselves be duped and brainwashed by patriarchal society? From being too timid and conventional? Feminist theologies of the erotic end up implying these characteristics about women who are still erotically oppressed. Mary McClintock Fulkerson, who has studied the experience of nonfeminist women who "fail" to see the sexism in scripture, points out the arrogant disregard of such feminist logic:

> We would have to assume that women who do not agree with [feminist] accounts are lobotomized by distorted discourse. Even an account that explains divergence by assuming women do not know

---

22. Ellison, *Erotic Justice*, 75.

how they are oppressed cannot be satisfied with the implication that women are rendered utterly passive as readers of the tradition.[23]

Short of being arrogant, the negative stance vis-à-vis tradition ends up producing a vacuum of interpretation around women's experience. The best feminist theologians of the erotic can say about women's pain and alienation is that their "true" experience is buried beneath layers of distortion. In these theologies, the meaning of women's testimony about their experiences of the erotic is simply assumed to be what women say it is — or else a lie generated by a woman's ignorance of her oppression. The content of what a woman names and claims is assumed to represent the "truth" — as opposed to what tradition tells the woman, which is usually assumed to be false. But this begs the question of what can ever be taken as "true" in experience (or, for that matter, in tradition). As Fulkerson says, "My quarrel is with the notion that our knowledge of ourselves is the essentially correct reflection, a mimesis, of our real and true selves."[24] She does not conclude that experience is worthless or that appeals to it can never be made. Rather, appeals must be acknowledged as limited and contextual.[25] Their content rarely stands on its own without interpretation.

The use of experience in theology is more like the use of raw data in science than like evidence in a proof; experience always needs to be contextualized and interpreted before drawing conclusions, which is certainly true of any individual woman's experience. Therefore, a better way to use women's experience for doing sexual ethics would be to assume that the erotic experiences women testify to need further interpretation. They are the ongoing construction sites in which certain meanings of the erotic are being configured and reconfigured. Women's testimonies reflect contexts in which the erotic is being produced; their testimonies need to be deciphered further. Instead of saying, "If so many women experience x, that must prove some profound truth," we should simply say, "If so many women experience x, we should be suspicious. We must figure out what is keeping things that way."

Making the kind of break Ellison talks about, after all — clearly and definitively breaking away from "old" ways of thinking — is not at all easy.

23. Fulkerson, *Changing the Subject,* 57.
24. Fulkerson, *Changing the Subject,* 27.
25. Fulkerson, *Changing the Subject,* 57.

As we shall see, many ordinary girls and young women repeat traditional and even stereotypical ideas about the erotic over and over again. They find it difficult to grasp new ways of thinking about it, though not for lack of trying. Girls and women are not brainwashed or duped, nor are they all timid. Most are struggling to create for themselves meaningful and wholesome erotic lives. They are frustrated by their own inability to figure out the meaning of the erotic and by the very stereotypes and traps into which they find themselves falling.

We need therefore to ask how "distorted" or traditional attitudes about femininity and the erotic become so deeply lodged under the skin. This study focuses on adolescent girls since they are a group most vulnerable to influence and perhaps least capable of independently creating new meanings. We shall ask the following sorts of questions: Why do girls still give up on themselves erotically, despite years of feminist attempts at empowering them? Why do girls seek the same stereotypical types of erotic relationships even after discovering them to be neither good nor satisfying? What happens in girls' lives to explain why generation after generation of them comply with what boys want and find this compliance "erotic"?

In the coming pages, we explore in detail the various difficulties teenage girls face in the expression of their eroticism. For now, we may briefly note how these difficulties challenge the theology we have been discussing. If we dismiss the misery and perplexity girls and women can experience, we simply label it "false" or "wrong," thus leaving ourselves without adequate ways to understand it. We do not wish to affirm the erotic confusion and romantic obsession, for example, to which girls are prone. Just as Fulkerson does not necessarily affirm nonfeminist women's benign readings of scripture, we do not have to conclude that girls' erotic behavior is always salutary. We are not forced to conclude that girls' way of thinking about the erotic is just as good as the way feminist theologians of the erotic think about it. Girls' experiences may indeed be unfortunate, but they are not false. They cry out for interpretation.

Women's Experience as Divine?

Davaney's final point is that feminist theologians have tended to do such a charitable reading of women's experience that they have drawn overly simple correspondences between it and God's purpose for human life. "While often simultaneously granting the contingency of its arguments and the plurality and diversity of its referents, feminist theology pleaded its normative case on the felicitous coincidence of female nature or experience, tradition, and divine purpose."[26] Such feminist theology appears to assume that women have some special access to divine wisdom by virtue of their being women. This might seem preposterous were we not to recall once again that the goal of any experiential feminism, like a feminist theology of the erotic, is to provide a better, more adequate vision than the one produced by androcentric, patriarchal theology. For too long, traditional theologies have drawn implicit correspondences between divinity and maleness, divine purpose and male experience. To correct this, reflecting on the divine from a female perspective has been necessary, emphasizing the blessing God places on experiences that are uniquely female and reorienting theological thinking by taking those experiences seriously into account.

Nevertheless, the risk here is of invoking God's blessing upon experiences that might not be deserving of it. As we learned in the previous chapter, feminist theologians of the erotic sometimes equate the erotic with the sacred. They argue that God is known through erotic, and even specifically sexual, experiences. Again, such arguments are primarily mounted to counter traditional assumptions about the relationship between sexuality and the sacred. As Plaskow asks plaintively: "Can we stop evicting our sexuality from the synagogue . . . ?" She is realistic enough to acknowledge that sexuality is not automatically or by definition sacred. "The unification of sexuality and spirituality is a sometime gift, a measure of the possible, rather than a reality of everyday."[27] Other feminist theologians of the erotic are less restrained, however.

Feminist theological discourse about the erotic is sometimes naive, not only in its invocation of the sacred but also in its descriptions of erotic relationship. These theologians want us to believe that erotic relationships are the most natural thing in the world and that good ones come easily once one achieves the right mind-set and respects the norm of mutuality. They affirm an authentic, natural Eros that will surface to act as its own moral guide. But evidence suggests that erotic relationships are not necessarily natural and do not always come easily. In fact, truly fulfilling erotic relationships appear to be rather rare, especially for adolescents.

---

26. Davaney, "Continuing the Story but Departing the Text," 202.
27. Plaskow, *Standing Again at Sinai*, 207.

Adolescents often have difficulty doing right by each other in the sexual realm. Their erotic relationships are often painfully far from the vision feminist theologians of the erotic would promote. Adolescents need more than a bit of courage and a reminder about mutuality to achieve sexual relationships that embody what these theologies profess.

Implications for a Sexual Ethic for Adolescents

Given these challenges to the confident logic of feminist theologies of the erotic, embracing a degree of skepticism regarding the possibilities of Eros where adolescents are concerned would seem wise. We must do so, however, without returning to a discourse of danger and suspicion. Adolescents have heard enough warnings. A sexual ethic for adolescents must consist of something other than prohibition, even if they are among the most vulnerable when sexually active. *Today's adolescents need clues about how to achieve fulfilling relationships even when the meaning of sexuality is unsettled and they cannot exercise full confidence in it.* The unsettled status of sexuality is, for better or worse, the context in which today's adolescents are coming of age. They live "between worlds," as Weeks put it, and amidst changing expectations. If they are to engage in erotic relationships that have any stability and purpose, they need some practical guidance as well as a more chastened, serious approach.

Accordingly, the rest of this study proceeds as follows. First, I consider some evidence that erotic relationships are far from liberatory for many contemporary adolescent girls. Suspicious of the common experience this evidence reveals, I then turn to psychological and psychoanalytic theories to interpret it. Finally, I sketch an alternative to feminist theologies of the erotic based on the possibilities of trust within an atmosphere of vulnerability.

This sort of sober approach befits the complexity of human erotic experience and respects the difficulty many young people have with it. While sobering, the approach is not necessarily negative. Once we no longer expect all erotic relationships to be paradisaical, we can begin to seek pragmatic ways to build the best ones we can. Once we no longer strive for the Eros of Eden, we can attempt to construct moral norms for the real world.

FOUR

Listening to Adolescent Girls
Voice the Erotic

> Once more there is a question which gives me no peace: "Is it right? Is it right
> that I should have yielded so soon, that I am so ardent, just as ardent and eager
> as Peter himself? May I, as a girl, let myself go to this extent?" ... I am afraid
> of myself, I am afraid that in my longing I am giving myself too quickly.
> — Anne Frank, *The Diary of Anne Frank*

THE QUESTIONS WE ASK OURSELVES about sex and love are often
tortured ones. Adolescents, in particular, often seem overwhelmed
with angst. Their distress stymies many adults and, were they to admit
it, many adolescents as well, but if we consider the many challenges adolescents face, especially at the dawn of the twenty-first century when the
status of sexuality is contested, their distress makes sense. In this book
thus far, I have maintained that theologians and ethicists who concentrate
on defending or promoting the value of Eros represent a valuable voice
within sexual ethics but an insufficient one for the problems of adolescent sexuality. Their overconfidence in the erotic is unwarranted, and their
heavy reliance on a discourse of liberation from repression is ultimately
inadequate. Similarly, by focusing on the virtue of relationality, they tend
to miss the real problems adolescents have.

This chapter will begin the process of interpreting adolescent distress
about sexuality and the erotic by listening closely to accounts that adolescent girls themselves offer. These accounts strongly suggest that girls
today are still significantly troubled about naming and claiming their
erotic desires. They show that feminist theologians' confidence in the
erotic is premature. Girls are pained and confused in a way that goes
beyond lack of enlightenment or failure of courage. For them, the erotic
is not so much repressed — it could presumably be made to surface given
sufficient encouragement and support — as their gender disempowers

84

them. This condition is reflected in the awkward and even troubling ways they voice the erotic. Their stories illustrate the need to move beyond a discourse of liberating the erotic to a more practical ethic of erotic relationship.

As this chapter shows, some girls have trouble reconciling being erotic and being female. The world they inhabit offers precious few satisfying and wholesome ways to be both. Eros and femaleness are constructed as incompatible. Unless this world were to change, therefore, *un*repressed eroticism would still not represent a solution. Their problems, in other words, are not the focus of feminist theologians of the erotic: That these girls need to overcome their shame of passion is not as significant as that they are truly ambivalent. Often they have little if any conception of themselves as erotic to begin with, that is, of ever becoming passionate or sexual beings. These girls fear talking about their erotic desires, but even more they are silent because they cannot decide what those desires mean and whether they are entitled to them. No one with whom they can identify has voiced or modeled eroticism for them. Other girls can imagine eroticism, but their imagination is sadly limited. If these girls use the term "erotic" at all, they simply refer to their longing to be girlfriends and wives, which is their experience of Eros. The ideal of being attached to someone as part of a couple absorbs them, becoming their primary if not exclusive "erotic" dream. The erotic is subtly but effectively constructed for them as that yearning to be a girlfriend — so that "erotic" simply stands for this desire. Their eroticism is not repressed per se but narrowly defined as romantic longing. Either way, these problems are ultimately problems of power — the powerlessness of their gender — not problems of repression.

Feminist theologians of the erotic could probably offer an explanation for girls' erotic silence. They would likely argue that girls' silence represents a falsity that must be broken by those who know the truth and are willing to speak it.[1] This explanation is dissatisfactory for reasons I

---

1. Feminist theologians are not the only ones who rely on such a discourse. On the morning after Barbara Walters's celebrated interview with Monica Lewinsky, *Good Morning America* invited a Catholic priest and a rabbi to share their opinions of what Ms. Lewinsky had said about her affair with President Clinton. Specifically, they were asked to comment on Ms. Lewinsky's reference to the president's religious beliefs. She had characterized Bill Clinton as deeply torn between expressing his sensuality and holding fast to his religious convictions. Immediately the priest said, "That dichotomy is false. Sexuality is a good gift of God's creation."

I may not have said anything different were I given thirty seconds to speak on national television. Nevertheless, for people who want to think seriously about sex and religion, the answer

have already given and about which I say more later. But for now, let us consider how girls' tendency to conflate the erotic with romantic longing might look from their theological perspective. Feminist theologians of the erotic could probably inspire girls to dream other dreams, which would be positive and helpful. Girls need to know that being "feminine" includes not only romance, but also independence, self-definition, creativity, and passion. But feminist theological discourse about the erotic strongly implies that nonfeminist desires like romantic longing are disingenuous expressions of the erotic. The implication is that a girl who gives in to this longing and finds it erotic has been misled and has yet to see the light. Insofar as feminist theologies of the erotic inspire girls to reach for new definitions of girlhood, they are helpful; but insofar as they rely on enlightenment discourse, they miss an opportunity to probe more deeply the magnetism that romance holds for many young women.

As I demonstrate in this chapter and the next, what adolescent girls need instead of feminist admonishing is being understood on their own terms. We should not assume that girls are all the same; at the same time, we need to figure out why a lot of them eroticize romance. Ultimately, adolescent girls need something besides more frequent invitations to name and claim their experience. They deserve to hear from feminists that both their ambivalence and their inclination toward romance are understandable — if not always in their best interest — and that historical and psychological reasons exist to explain both. This communication can be accomplished without telling girls that they are "naturally" more relational than boys, and without necessarily celebrating this gender difference. These approaches fail to address a set of deeply rooted and intertwined issues about gender, sex, and power. Girls deserve instead sustained and thoughtful theorizing about what taking a gendered journey through adolescence actually means.

---

is ultimately unsatisfying. As theologians, we must acknowledge and contend with the fact that whether or not we think sexuality and religion are theoretically compatible, many others still experience them as incompatible. Calling their experiences false does not help. We must acknowledge the role that theology and the church have historically played in fostering that dichotomy. We must also acknowledge that theologians continue to construct sex and religion in ways that feed the dichotomy — for example, when we continually choose examples of asceticism to model selflessness. We must figure out what status we are really willing to give sensual pleasure. And we must acknowledge that sexuality may not always be a good gift, as when the man who occupies the nation's highest office appears unable to stop at flirtation.

The Difficulty of Finding Adolescent Voices

Listening to adolescent voices helps keep grounded in reality our interpretation of adolescent sexuality. Finding adequate resources for this task, however, is not easy, for at least four reasons. First, we do not simply need to gather yet more empirical evidence of teenagers' confusion and poor judgment about sexual behavior; we already have this data in abundance. What we are really after is how teenagers attempt to resolve their own distress about sexuality and the erotic. How well are they able to decide the meanings of sex and femininity? How much confidence can they muster? In their perception, what is hard about being young and female and faced with decisions about their sexuality? Ideally, what we need are researchers who are interested in these questions and who actually talk to girls and ask girls what they think. Such studies, however, do not abound. Few psychologists directly ask teenagers what they think. They do not, by and large, ask adolescent girls to reflect on their experiences of sexuality and the erotic. Instead, researchers ask questions that produce the following kinds of data: correlations between the frequency of sexual behavior (especially intercourse) with age, family structure, and other demographic features; correlations between contraceptive use and the same factors; and levels of "permissiveness" among adolescents with respect to sexual behavior. Such studies produce important findings, but they do not probe the underlying experiences. They do not, for example, tell us why girls define the erotic in terms of romance. They do not tell us what girls think about the role gender plays in their experiences.

A second, closely related reason for the inadequacy of most recent psychological research lies in its methodology. The voice of distress is most likely to emerge in the context of open-ended interviews, yet most researchers employ forced-choice questionnaires.[2] Forced-choice questions always produce answers. But for our purposes, more revelatory responses

---

2. The researcher devises a set of questions for which the subjects either choose among a set of answers or rank answers on a scale. Empirical results thus take the form of quantitative data about sexuality. I do not mean simply that studies aim only for quantitative information about sexuality (e.g., "x is the median age at which these girls first engaged in intercourse"), but that even information about the quality of sexuality is presented quantitatively (e.g., "x number of girls said they felt comfortable talking to their parents about sex as opposed to y number who did not"). From this kind of research, we gain only a statistical impression of adolescent sexuality, and at that, one that the researcher frames from the outset. Study subjects create neither their own responses nor, of course, the questions they will answer. See Susan Moore and Doreen Rosenthal for a critique of this kind of psychological research into adolescent sexuality. "The Social Context of Adolescent Sexuality: Safe Sex Implications," in *Journal of Adolescence* 15 (1992): 416.

are, on the one hand, the dead-ends, gaps, and contradictions exposed in girls' speech when they try to articulate their erotic experience and, on the other hand, the reasons girls themselves offer for why they are not capable of supplying better answers. We can hear such responses only if girls are allowed to identify their own questions and struggle toward their own answers without the benefit of options generated and supplied by the researcher. If we want to know how and why the erotic is a problem for girls, the methodology of most research limits its value for us.

Demonstrating distress and perplexity is, of course, harder than demonstrating confidence and clarity. As Catharine MacKinnon has said, by itself silence is not eloquent.[3] A third reason, then, for the difficulty in finding empirical information about adolescent experiences of the erotic is simply the elusiveness of our prize. If girls experience difficulty voicing the erotic — which is our working hypothesis — then by definition they are unlikely to be able to articulate their own difficulty doing so. Therefore, sometimes we have to work backward from what girls do not say to understand the conflicts in what they do say. Imagining what their discourse might be like if girls voiced the erotic without difficulty maybe helpful. We can imagine a variety of expressions — possibility, longing, anticipation, excitement, relief, disgust, joy, and more — that narrators who felt free and confident expressing eroticism might use to describe it. The erotic might mean different things to different girls. Only against this hypothetical variety does the shallowness of girls' actual discourse become more apparent (and therefore more theoretically interesting).

A fourth and final explanation for the dearth of resources on our topic is that much of the available research in the field of psychology is limited to specific populations. The research tends to focus narrowly on the roots of "problematic" sexual behavior — the behaviors that cause teenage pregnancy and sexually transmitted disease — and therefore addresses populations with high rates of pregnancy and disease. Studies focus even more particularly on poor and working-class girls whose pregnancies and diseases are deemed especially troublesome.

----

3. She is writing about the difficulty of proving how pornography harms women: "That pornography chills women's expression is difficult to demonstrate empirically because silence is not eloquent." Catharine MacKinnon, *Toward a Feminist Theory of the State* (Cambridge, Mass.: Harvard University Press, 1989), 206.

Narratives on Adolescent Sexuality

Since much of the psychological research on adolescent female sexuality is not directly useful for this book's project, I turn beyond the field of psychology to other work that is relevant to the issues that concern us. I turn primarily to the field of journalism. In recent years, several feminist writers have completed participant-observer studies of female adolescence. They have met and interviewed scores of girls, each bringing to her work the analytical skills of their respective disciplines. I draw most heavily upon Sharon Thompson and Peggy Orenstein, and to a lesser extent upon Patricia Hersch and Leora Tanenbaum and others. What these writers all share are commitments to feminist research principles and transforming the lives of girls. In one way or another, they all try to shed light on girls' struggles, including, at least implicitly, struggles with the erotic. Their methodologies incorporate open-ended interviews that give subjects wide latitude to talk about their own experiences using their own words. What Thompson, Orenstein, and others have produced, in effect, is a body of female adolescent *narratives* about sexuality and the erotic.

This body of narratives is also useful to us because of the diversity of girls interviewed. Collectively, the narratives represent adolescents from poor, working-class, and middle-class communities; from urban and suburban areas of the country; and of white, African-American, and Hispanic backgrounds. Some were pregnant; some were mothers. Most were heterosexual, but some were lesbian. (At times, differences in identity appear to make a difference in erotic experience, and when possible, these differences are noted.) Through the writers' reconstructions of conversations with girls, we can hear what girls have to say when asked to weave their own accounts. But before turning to these narratives, considering the aims and methods used would be helpful. I will provide brief overviews of the different research projects and also caution readers regarding some of their limits.

As social historian, writer, and activist, Sharon Thompson has based her work upon extensive interviewing with adolescent (primarily working-class) girls. In a long-term study conducted between 1978 and 1986, Thompson interviewed over four hundred adolescents, gathering their accounts of their experiences of sex, romance, and pregnancy.[4] Thompson

---

4. Sharon Thompson, "Search for Tomorrow: Feminism and the Reconstruction of Teen Romance," in *Pleasure and Danger: Exploring Female Sexuality,* ed. Carole S. Vance (Boston:

describes the historical period about which she writes as "the brief but amazing period in the history of sex, gender, and adolescence when [girls] knew of almost no reason *not* to have sex"[5] — the period of the late 1970s through the mid-1980s that came after the legalization of contraception and abortion but before the AIDS outbreak.[6] As I noted in chapter 1, adolescents' understanding of the meaning of sex had shifted significantly prior to this period and continued to shift during it. Hence, Thompson unearthed a great deal of anguish and perplexity with regard to sexuality, romance, and sexual desiring.

The main drawback to Thompson's work is that she too readily types the girls she spoke to, dividing them into categories such as "Victims of Love" and "Romantic Strategists." She may do this to underscore the point that girls themselves are all too happy to adopt roles and conduct themselves according to "scripts" about sex, love, and romance. Clearly, however, Thompson's device also risks reinforcing those same roles and scripts, implying that roles are deterministic and that any given individual can fall into only one "type." Thompson's categorization also prevents readers from drawing their own conclusions about the narratives.

Peggy Orenstein is a journalist whose work has appeared in the *New York Times, Mother Jones,* and *Vogue.* She has written primarily about gender, childhood, beauty myths, and reproductive freedom. Her work addresses the impact dominant society and culture have on girls' and women's identity and experience. In a book-length study, *SchoolGirls: Young Women, Self-Esteem, and the Confidence Gap,* Orenstein investigates several of the reasons for the long-standing problem that girls' sense of self-esteem diminishes during adolescence. She notes the puzzling contradiction between abundant evidence of women's liberation and remaining deficits in adolescent girls' self-esteem:

In spite of the changes in women's roles in society, in spite of the changes in their own mothers' lives, many of today's girls fall

Routledge & Kegan Paul, 1984), 350–84; "Putting a Big Thing into a Little Hole: Teenage Girls' Accounts of Sexual Initiation," in *Journal of Sex Research* 27, no. 3 (August 1990): 341–61; and *Going All the Way: Teenage Girls' Tales of Sex, Romance, and Pregnancy* (New York: Hill and Wang, 1995).

5. Thompson, *Going All the Way,* 11.

6. This period of recent history is treated here as contemporary, as I contend that adolescents still wrestle with most of these same questions, and many of the same problems remain. (AIDS has proved to be the most significant historical intervention, but study of its effects on the erotic is beyond the scope of this book.)

into traditional patterns of low self-image, self-doubt, and self-censorship of their creative and intellectual potential. Although all children experience confusion and a faltering sense of self at adolescence, girls' self-regard drops further than boys' and never catches up. They emerge from their teenage years with reduced expectations and have less confidence in themselves and their abilities than do boys.[7]

Orenstein's explicit focus in this study is self-esteem, and her interview data sheds light on certain contradictions and problems that are closely related to it, including eroticism. To immerse herself in teenage life for this study, Orenstein spent the 1992–93 academic year as an observer in two California middle schools, attending classes and extracurricular activities.[8] Among the classes she observed were sessions in sexuality education. Orenstein also visited the homes of several of the girls she met and became acquainted with their families, providing her with ample opportunity to observe boys and girls in informal settings outside the classroom. As a result of her research, Orenstein was able to document the state of adolescent gender relations. Many of her interviews covered the topics of sex, love, and romance. Orenstein also explicitly invited her interviewees to speculate on how gender difference affected their experiences in these regards. This approach adds value to her study from our perspective.

Patricia Hersch also went back to school. She is a journalist who has been published in several newspapers and magazines, including the *Washington Post* and *McCalls*. She was a contributing editor to *Psychology Today* and has studied homeless teenagers for the National Institute of Drug Abuse and Georgetown University Child Development Center. Between 1992 and 1995, Hersch attended an elementary school, a middle school, and a high school in Reston, Virginia, a planned community outside of

---

7. Peggy Orenstein, *SchoolGirls: Young Women, Self-Esteem, and the Confidence Gap* (New York: Bantam Doubleday Dell Publishing Group, 1994), xvi. This study was explicitly designed as a follow-up to the 1990 American Association of University Women's report *Shortchanging Girls, Shortchanging America*. The AAUW had studied the way American public schools treat girls and boys differently, producing results that surprised many people, including journalists like Orenstein. The report analyzed gender differences in competence, and perceptions of competence, in academic disciplines such as math and science. The study showed that while girls performed as well as or better than boys in these areas, they were less confident in their performance. American Association of University Women, *Shortchanging Girls, Shortchanging America: Full Data Report* (Washington, D.C.: American Association of University Women, 1990).

8. Weston School is a suburban school serving mostly white students from a diversity of class backgrounds. Audubon Middle School is an urban school serving poor and working-class students of ethnic minorities.

Washington, D.C. She conducted interviews outside of school with approximately sixty teenagers whose parents had given her permission to talk to them in complete confidence. These interviews were conducted over the course of several years, yielding a longitudinal perspective. Eight of these sixty teenagers she chose as representative narrators and followed their lives up until 1997. She published her book, *A Tribe Apart: A Journey into the Heart of American Adolescence,* in 1998.

Leora Tanenbaum interviewed fifty women and girls between the ages of fourteen and sixty-six for her book, *Slut! Growing up Female with a Bad Reputation.* She defines labeling a girl a "slut" as an act of sexual harassment and seeks to examine the phenomenon of slut-bashing from both a historical and contemporary perspective.

The open-ended interview methodology used by Thompson, Orenstein, Hersch, and Tanenbaum has drawbacks. They all present their findings in nonscientific journalistic prose; readers cannot examine the data themselves. We do not, in other words, have access through their work to the uninterrupted narratives of the interviewees but only to interpretations of those narratives. Occasionally, in fact, one suspects that the writers' interpretive frameworks are constructed in ways that may misrepresent the girls' original intent. Nevertheless, their work is still preferable to the other available research. To gain from it, we turn now to content — that is, to the adolescent girls themselves, their stories, and the researchers' interpretations of them.

Voicing the Erotic

What do teenage girls say when they are invited to talk about and interpret their erotic experiences? The invitation intimidates many girls, and they hesitate as if to consider the implications of any answer they might give. They also respond to the invitation with seriousness and intensity. Despite this reaction (or perhaps even because of it), girls' answers are often complex.

Disavowing Sexual Desire

Some girls seem to sense the freight erotic desiring carries and clearly resist the very idea of characterizing themselves as erotic. One sixteen-year-old girl expresses the quandary of being a sexually excited female:

> I don't know how to bring up the subject of these feelings I get.
> Girls aren't supposed to — they're not supposed to get excited. I
> know my brother does. I mean, he plays with himself. It's hard to
> know what to think about this subject. I wake up, and I've had a
> dream and I'm all excited because of the dream, I think. So then my
> body starts moving on me. Do you know what I mean? I'm not sure
> I do, myself! I'm sorry I can't write better. I mean, express myself.[9]

This girl was a patient of psychiatrist Robert Coles, who has studied
children and adolescents for many years. She had written a letter to him,
comparing herself with her twin brother. He included excerpts from her
letter in his commentary on a survey of teenage sexual behavior conducted
by *Rolling Stone* magazine in the early 1980s. This patient's letter, and her
sending of it, actually reveals remarkable self-awareness, and yet she claims
to be unsure of what she has said and even unsure of what she has felt.
When trying to express something that they believe they ought not even
know about, many girls make false starts and appear confused. This one
experiences feelings of excitement that directly contradict her belief that
"girls aren't supposed to get excited." Two tangible results of this conflict
are self-doubt and incoherence: "Do you know what I mean? I'm not sure
I do, myself! I'm sorry I can't write better. I mean, express myself."

Because girls often acknowledge that they do experience erotic feelings,
their inability to express them does not necessarily spring from physical
immaturity or simple lack of interest. Undoubtedly, for some teenage
girls, not being able to say much about the erotic simply means that the
erotic is not yet part of their lives. But for others, the problem is staying
with the troubling feelings they have long enough to talk about them.
This precise conflict causes distress, uncertainty, and hesitation.

The conflict may cause girls to dissociate from their feelings. As soon
as this girl mentioned that her "body started moving on her," she claimed
not to know what such "movement" really meant. Perhaps she simply
experienced a loss of control brought on by new and unfamiliar sensations,
and now she voices that loss of control by claiming ignorance. But she
may also be genuinely perturbed by her bodily feelings. If she eventually
ceased even acknowledging their existence and became alienated from her
own embodied experience, that outcome would be unfortunate indeed.

---

9. Robert Coles, *Sex and the American Teenager* (New York: Harper Collins Books, 1985), 4.

Sensing the Double Standard

Gender often lies behind a girl's questioning her entitlement to sexual desire. Anne Frank, whose famous and anguished autobiographical account of adolescent desire began this chapter, grasped that her being a girl made a difference: "May I, as a girl, let myself go to this extent?" She questioned whether she was supposed to be as ardent and eager as her boyfriend, Peter. And yet her question caused her to doubt herself, not Peter. She even admits that she is afraid of herself.

While some girls, like Robert Coles's patient, are caught in the trap of lacking enough trust in themselves to be sure of their feelings, other girls are caught in a different trap. They may experience erotic desires and actually want to act on them but feel that doing so would conflict with their internalized belief that girls ought to fend off sexual advances. In other words, they fear a double standard will be applied against them.

On the one hand, there are girls who wish to act on their desires but not to the same extent as their boyfriends do. They may enjoy kissing and other sexual activities but do not want to engage in intercourse. One girl in Patricia Hersch's study, Courtney, falls into this category.

> One night when Dee comes over, Courtney and she have their millionth discussion about sex. While the noise of the television drones in the background, they munch on M&M's and grapes. They go over the same ground as if it is new. Dee starts, "I haven't had sex yet, but hopefully I will love him."
>
> "Yeah," says Courtney. "You've got to be sure they're smart enough to know about a girl's body."
>
> "Right," says Dee. "You don't want to have sex with someone stupid."
>
> "I told you I didn't know where this was leading with Nat," says Courtney with a sigh. "I don't know if it's going to lead to sex. I'm not sure."
>
> "I think a lot of teenagers are stupid," says Dee, trying to make her friend's decision easier. "They think everyone's having sex so you have to too. A lot of people are having sex, but not that many. Personally, I don't think I'm mature enough to have sex anyway. I'm not comfortable enough with my body, let alone theirs, to have sex."
>
> "The thing is," says Courtney, "I know I'd get so mad if I had sex with a guy and then they didn't speak to me again. I know I'd

probably prefer them not to have sex with me at this stage in my life." She is ashamed of not wanting to have sex, thinking it shows how immature she is. She goes back and forth about Nat as her first partner.[10]

It sounds as though Courtney and Dee have heard at least part of the message that feminist theologians of the erotic are sending — that they deserve physical pleasure and therefore sexual partners who understand the female body. They can say all the right things about needing to feel comfortable with their bodies and being mature about physical intimacy. Yet, in the end, these do not really seem to be the issues. Courtney sounds more concerned that Nat will not speak to her after she has sex with him. "The thing is, I know I'd get so mad if I had sex with a guy and then they didn't speak to me again." She hints at the knowledge that boys are frequently just interested in intercourse and break up with girls once they have had it.

On the other hand, there are girls who claim not to mind sexual intercourse and some who enjoy it. Nevertheless, they still feel odd or wrong for having these desires. The classic double standard for sexual activity — that is, the age-old assumption that boys' sexual activity is tolerated and even encouraged while people frown upon girls' sexual activity — still exists. Girls' sexual activity carries more negative social consequences, and hence some girls deeply fear the future consequences to themselves of giving in to desire. One sixteen-year-old girl voiced the double standard this way:

> Girls who are sexually active, especially if they don't hide it, they're seen as cheap or easy. Guys be like, you know, "I'm gonna see what I can get. You done her? Yeah, I done her, too." And adults look down on you when you're a sexually active teen, like, they never did it when they were young too, right?[11]

As this girl suggests, adults enforce the double standard as harshly as do teenagers. Sometimes they can be quite cruel. One of Tanenbaum's interviewees recalls the day that the principal of her school implicitly accused her of being a slut.

---

10. Patricia Hersch, *A Tribe Apart: A Journey into the Heart of American Adolescence* (New York: Ballantine Books, 1998), 175.

11. Lynn Phillips, ed., *The Girls Report: What We Know and Need to Know about Growing Up Female* (New York: National Council for Research on Women, 1998), 34.

When I was a senior in high school, in 1990, I was called out of class and told to go to the principal's office. He walked me out to the back of the school, where it was spray-painted Pam Is A Slut. I was the only Pam in the school. It was on the whole back of the school building, in huge letters, facing the soccer field and the football field.

He asked me, "Do you know who would do this?" There was no preparation. There was no concern, no compassion for me. No, "How are you?" Just: "Do you know who would do this?" I didn't know it was there until he showed it to me. It was awful. He was very accusatory about it, like, "What did you do wrong that would make somebody do this?" I remember thinking, "I don't know who would do this; why are you asking me?" I just walked away. I remember crying in the bathroom and crying to a few girls. I felt that I was being branded for something that had happened to me, as if I were responsible. The writing had to be sandblasted off.[12]

One effect of the double standard is that girls receive no positive concept of female eroticism. They simply are not presented with images of sexually desiring girls or women. "'In the media, sex is always up to the boy,' complains fourteen-year-old Lauren. . . . 'It's a very rare occasion on TV when there's a boy who does not want to have sex. You also don't see a girl who wants sex as much as the boy does.'"[13] Girls often report that parents overreact to mentions of sex, assuming either that their daughters are obsessed with sex or headed for danger. They seem unable to entertain the notion that their daughters might simply have a healthy interest in sex.

"You don't tell your parents about sex," says Dee. "They just freak out. If you tell them, they think you're a whore or something."

They are so contradictory, says Courtney. "If you tell them that you're not ready to have sex they conclude, 'Oh God, sex is on their mind. They're trying to cover up for it.' They get hysterical. If you tell them that you think you are ready, they're like, 'You're not going out tonight.'"[14]

---

12. Leora Tanenbaum, *Slut! Growing Up Female with a Bad Reputation* (New York: Seven Stories Press, 1999), 102–5.
13. Tanenbaum, *Slut!* 117.
14. Hersch, *A Tribe Apart,* 175–76.

It follows that parents who cannot imagine their daughter's eroticism also cannot share images of female eroticism with their daughters.

The double standard does a poor job of enforcing moral norms for female adolescent sexual behavior. It cannot rule specific behaviors out because, after all, it permits those same behaviors in boys. Instead, the double standard just makes girls feel that they themselves are morally bad. It attacks girls' sense of self.

> I started kissing neighborhood boys in fourth grade. At this point I was still a "good girl." By sixth grade it got more into fooling around. And then by eighth grade it was everything but intercourse. I definitely enjoyed it. I had physical pleasure. But at the same time I felt that it was wrong, and that there was something wrong with me. Not that what I was doing was wrong, or that there was something wrong with the guys, but that *I* was wrong.[15]

In short, the gendered double standard for sexual behavior ensures that adolescent girls are poorly equipped to find meaning in their erotic experiences. They are left with few positive ideas about female erotic behavior. For that matter, they are left with few ideas about what might be genuinely wrong with their behavior either ("not that [I felt] what I was doing was wrong"). They just think something is wrong with them. They are left with no guidance for recognizing either good or bad erotic experiences. Instead, they tend to distance themselves from the erotic altogether.

Fearing Vulnerability

Other reasons exist as well for the distance girls place between themselves and their erotic feelings. Girls often watch other girls become so distracted by romantic involvement that they drop out of school. As a savvy girl named Dashelle observes: "Girls want boyfriends and all that little mess, but to me, I think boys distract you from school and everything. They can knock things out of your mind. So I don't want a boyfriend."[16]

In other instances, girls fear that if they open themselves up to erotic feelings, they might also make themselves vulnerable to sexual violence and sexually transmitted disease. For many girls, becoming sexually involved with boys is a genuinely dangerous proposition about which they have

---

15. Tanenbaum, *Slut!* 105.
16. Orenstein, *SchoolGirls*, 237–38.

been well warned by their friends and sisters, not to mention the adults in their lives. Often, girls who are economically or ethnically marginalized fear that violence and disease will be the price of desiring. They have watched sexually active sisters and girlfriends be victimized, so they do not let themselves become interested in sex. Other girls, especially those who are poor and belong to communities that discourage abortion, additionally perceive that becoming sexually involved with boys leads to a future of early motherhood and continued poverty. Contrary to the popular perception that poor and working-class girls always *want* to get pregnant, many say things such as:

> I think that boyfriends could get in my way, though. You fall in love with a boy and then you don't want to do anything. You just do what he wants to do and then you do nothing. So I don't want to fall in love. I know a girl who went with her boyfriend when she was fifteen, and she got pregnant and that was it. You have to keep your eyes open, and you can't fall in love, that's important.[17]

In short, sex and romance appear to be dangerous territory to many girls and for many reasons they might understandably be tentative about naming and claiming eroticism — being sexual too often literally means being vulnerable.

Experiencing the Gender Gap

However we interpret these excerpts, one common theme running through all of them is difficult to ignore: Girls observe that for boys, adolescence is different. The power of gender is a clearly discernible subtext of these narratives, and boys are clearly perceived to have more power than girls. The power with which these narrators credit boys is social, rhetorical, and relational, if not necessarily physical. Boys are free to "get excited"; boys can "see what they can get"; boys are immune from blame; boys have the power to distract rather than be distracted; boys can get their girlfriends to do what they want to do until their girlfriends "do nothing" on their own. Perhaps the most graphic description of boys' power came from Dashelle, who said, "They can knock things out of your mind."

Girls are not always explicit about the gender gap in erotic life, but their stories refer to it even when they are not fully conscious of it. In

---

17. Orenstein, *SchoolGirls,* 237.

Orenstein's story of Evie and Bradley, for instance, the subtext is clear. Evie reports having been "in love" with Bradley during the sixth grade even though he consistently treated her poorly. She craved his attention. When she said she would not have sex with him, he ignored her. When he finally noticed her again at the end of the seventh grade, she initially said yes to his proposition. Although she was nervous, and worried about becoming a slut, she wanted Bradley desperately and tried to convince herself that she just needed to get over with having sex. As the time drew closer, however, she worried more. Evie knew that having sex would change her, as it had changed other girls. She told Orenstein that after girls had sex, they started dressing differently, more provocatively, and even wearing their hair differently. They expressed not only a worse image but a worse opinion of themselves. In the end Evie turned Bradley down.

> "I feel scummy," she says softly, fluffing the grass with her fingers. "Even though I didn't actually do it, I feel like a total slut inside. I feel like a slut for considering it. It damaged my personality and my opinion of myself. And if people knew, nothing would happen to him, but it would damage the way I was treated...." "I just wish I could forget it," she says, rolling over on her back. "It makes me feel so bad about myself. I'm ashamed of myself. I wish I could wipe the glass clean. Like if I had Windex for my soul."[18]

Determining from this story what Evie wanted (except that she wanted Bradley as her boyfriend) is difficult, and that is the point. Her own desires, whatever they were — whether to have sex or not to have sex — are obscured in the awful situation in which she finds herself. Her desire is beside the point. Evie is trapped between a rock and a hard place, between "knowing the price of saying no" and worrying that "if she had sex with Bradley [she would become] a slut." Either way, she loses — either a relationship she desperately wants or her reputation.

On the other hand, Bradley's apparent power to control every turn in the story is remarkable. His seeming power to rebuff her, and to make her feel like a damaged person just for considering sex with him, is what comes through unambiguously in this narrative. Evie's estimation of herself has changed dramatically despite the fact that she did not even have

18. Orenstein, *SchoolGirls*, 55.

sex; she merely considered it. The horror Evie feels overwhelmed by is, as Orenstein points out, horror over her thoughts, not her actions. She ultimately refused sex with Bradley, so her only "transgression" was contemplating it. Yet even the thought is so repelling to her that she feels she has to clean her soul. Meanwhile, as she astutely recognizes, the situation affected Bradley barely at all. Were other people to find out about the episode, as she points out, "nothing would happen to him."

The erotic power differential between boys and girls hurts girls.[19] Perhaps its most heartbreaking aspect is the damage potential to girls' sense of self. When girls like Evie lose their own sense of agency and self-respect — sometimes for several years during adolescence — when they become strange and alien even to themselves, eroticism becomes not only intimidating but destructive. We might be tempted to think that a girl like Evie is just being overdramatic in rendering her story. Such a conclusion, however, would underestimate the seriousness to a teenager of the "slut" category. Girls often believe that this reputation will ruin their lives forever; and while lifelong damage probably rarely occurs, reputations certainly have tangible and lasting effects upon adolescents, especially girls. Girls and boys quickly place each other in categories whose implications linger for some time. Being perceived as a slut means, for many a girl, forfeiting a sense of self-respect and happiness for a long time. One of the most common threats to sense of self in female adolescence is categorization as a slut, and no true counterpart to it occurs in male adolescence.

We might also be tempted to think that Evie greatly overvalued being Bradley's girlfriend and should have just given up on him. To expect this action, however, would be to underestimate the lure of "girlfriendhood" for many adolescents. Many of the girls who live in fear of being labeled "sluts" nevertheless do not fear it enough to avoid romantic involvement altogether, suggesting that the prospect of romantic relationship is a powerful motivator in female adolescence. If girls perceive and experience that having a boyfriend increases their worth, then they are unlikely to avoid a romantic relationship that makes them feel worthy and special. But, as we have seen, they pay a price.

---

19. The power differential may ultimately hurt boys, too, albeit in a different way. As the next chapter shows, boys are often at risk of becoming detached and distant figures even to people they care deeply about.

Lacking Power

From these stories, I conclude that many girls are distressed and bewildered about the erotic — even to the point of doubting themselves and what they know. We thus already have at least some evidence to suggest that the problems with Eros run more deeply than feminist theologians of the erotic envision. Those theologians who encourage us to correct our thinking about sex and develop a more positive attitude toward it seem to be mistaken, if these narratives are reliable. These girls do not, by and large, have faulty conceptions of sex. Indeed, their insights into the realities of sex and romance are sometimes excruciatingly astute. Thus, thinking more correctly about the erotic will not remedy the girls' distress. These girls are not so much mistaken as they are caught in the shifting paradigms for sexuality and femininity. On the one hand, they know about Eros and sex and even know that they deserve to experience erotic feelings; yet on the other hand, they believe that being erotic conflicts with being a girl. (In fact, insofar as they experience outright condemnation or ridicule for being erotic, girls' thinking about the erotic is quite accurate.) They are not so much unenlightened as they are powerless to change the conditions that produce those paradigms. Nor is the problem primarily attitudinal, so that developing a more liberated attitude toward sexuality and Eros would suffice.

The girls we have heard from voice a conflict — between the prospect of being an erotic person and skepticism about whether this activity is even possible and proper in the world as they know it. This conflict produces significant distress for girls. Girls are aware that they cannot figure out their sexuality. They know, if you will, what they do not know. They make excuses for their own seeming lack of clarity, which only reveals how aware they are of the bind they are in. If they do not always grasp the political dimensions of their situation, they do seem to sense, at least in some cases, that their confusion puts them out of touch with their selves and that something is profoundly wrong with that. Even girls seem to sense that their attitude toward sexuality does not primarily need changing as much as the larger, disempowering context in which they are becoming sexual beings.

I question whether these problems are ones of repression per se, at least if "repression" is understood as inhibition or socialized modesty. I think instead that the girls we have heard from lack the power and resources to resist constructions of femininity and sexuality that confine them. In many cases, they lack even a language to talk about a passion that is supposedly available to all persons by virtue of being human.

What are the consequences of lacking power and resources? One is diminished moral agency. The hesitancy and sense of bafflement voiced in these narratives do not bode well for responsible decision making about sexual activity. Girls who are as ambivalent as we have heard are unlikely to make good decisions, if they make them at all, about protecting themselves. They forfeit their own moral agency and fail to communicate to their partners clear decisions about sexual activity. One tangible expression of this failure is the way "no" and "yes" become blurred in girls' discourse about consent. Because these girls lack the freedom to state either their wishes or their refusals, consent and refusal become difficult to distinguish. This conclusion is not the same as saying that girls' "no" really means "yes," a charge sometimes leveled against girls. Girls who actually say "no" when they really mean "yes," as some undoubtedly do, are just engaging in a verbal ploy to obscure an otherwise clear choice. Under the condition of lacking free choice, however, neither "no" nor "yes" really means anything.

Girls' failure to communicate clear answers, whatever the reason, is apparent in the following conversation. A group of girls is discussing whether boys need sex more than girls do. The exchange is both candid and poignant.

"Yes," says a girl named Paula, who is holding a compact and applying lipstick. "I mean, maybe. No. I don't know."

"I say yes," says Helen decisively. "Boys get horny."

All the girls laugh at this.

"Yeah," Paula says, "but girls get horny, too. Maybe she wants to have sex, but she can't ask."

Marta . . . speaks for the first time. "Maybe if she wants to do it, she won't say so. But she'll kind of lead him on to do it instead. Girls do that sometimes. They say 'no,' but they don't really mean it."

"Yeah," says Alanna, "we're evil."[20]

---

20. Orenstein, *SchoolGirls*, 220.

Paula and Marta articulate clearly the bind in which girls find themselves. According to their experience, many girls want sex but cannot request it or even assent to it. Therefore girls say "no," but do not really mean this either, so both assent and dissent lose their meaning. Girls lose the agentic power to agree or disagree. Indeed, Orenstein takes this conversation as evidence of "how deeply the girls have disconnected from their own desires, how, amid the tangle of that submersion, they do not imagine consent as saying 'yes,' but as saying 'no' in a particular way."[21]

Studies about first intercourse also provide evidence that girls' agency diminishes. Sharon Thompson asked heterosexual adolescent girls about "their first time" with their boyfriends and reports hearing the same story of bewilderment and lack of forethought over and over again.[22] Girls claimed: "I don't know what came over me that night. I really don't. I mean, I can't really answer it. But it happened"; "I tell you, I don't know why or how I did it. Maybe I just did it unconsciously."[23] "It was just like — pssst, one minute here, the next minute it was there. It happened. That was it."[24] Girls often explained first sex to Thompson in terms of the inevitability of the circumstances rather than a decision made: "Uhm, probably if I would have had my eyes opened, I would have realized it was going to happen. . . . He was over here once and my parents weren't — home — and I didn't realize basically what I got myself into."[25] Presumably, these girls did not feel responsible for their actions because they did not experience themselves as having chosen sex — they just did it "unconsciously." To have chosen sexual activity is to admit, after all, to desiring it; but if desiring sexual activity is incompatible with beliefs girls hold about themselves, then the latter will often win out: "I'm telling you I did it unconsciously because I wouldn't do a thing like that."[26]

Another serious consequence of lacking power, a more philosophical one, is the enormous burden that sexuality becomes for girls, which is unfortunate because sexuality should not have to be so burdensome. Sexuality becomes a burden for girls in part because they feel pressured into

21. Orenstein, *SchoolGirls*, 220.
22. "'My first time,'" Thompson writes, "had become a staple in girls' oral tradition, but girls still had few conventions to draw on to open or develop the subject. In this study, most girls said that all their experienced friends told the 'same story' about first intercourse." "Putting a Big Thing into a Little Hole," 343.
23. Thompson, "Putting a Big Thing into a Little Hole," 343.
24. Thompson, *Going All the Way*, 30.
25. Thompson, "Putting a Big Thing into a Little Hole," 346.
26. Thompson, "Putting a Big Thing into a Little Hole," 344.

having to make decisions about it prematurely. One fourteen-year-old, whose boyfriend asks her constantly to have intercourse, says that she thinks she is too young to have to respond. Nevertheless, she feels the decision is an unavoidable one.

> I think fourteen definitely sounds young, but I think tenth grade is about average. I'm not really excited about it because I don't think many girls enjoy it their first time, and I think it will be painful. But it's something that you want to get over with. I think it's a little too young to come up in relationships, but it is coming up. It's something you have to face. I think you have to deal with it at fourteen, decide.[27]

Girls' burden and distress are unfortunate because sexuality is a good thing. Feminist theologies of the erotic are right about that statement, at least: Sexuality can be a positive, even glorious part of human relationship. To pass into adulthood torn and confused about sexuality is to jeopardize something of potentially great value and sustenance. Sexuality can bring vigor and happiness to human life. If the evidence offered thus far is accurate, however, quite a few girls may not discover these qualities for some time. Imagine the chances for future joy if one's first and indelible impressions of sex resemble those reported to Thompson: "It didn't really hurt. It hurt a little bit. It was uncomfortable. I was pretty bored actually. I didn't see anything very nice about it." "It wasn't that I didn't like it. It was just kind of a letdown." "It wasn't really that good. There was nothing I really liked about it." "Oh, why would they even bother to leave that out of the movies?"[28]

Living for Love

So far, we have heard primarily from girls whose experience comprises perplexity about what "the erotic" means, noticeable reluctance to satisfy any of their erotic longings, and a fundamental lack of certainty about whether they should feel "erotic" at all. However, another set of experiences, apparently just as common during adolescence, appears at first to contradict all that angst. Some girls tell stories about their erotic ex-

27. Hersch, *A Tribe Apart,* 177.
28. Thompson, "Putting a Big Thing into a Little Hole," 346.

periences within romantic relationship with anything but reticence and distress. They seem adept and comfortable talking about how they became girlfriends and at times even sound obsessed with the topic. When explicitly asked to talk about romance or love rather than Eros or sex (and even sometimes when they are asked to talk about sex), many girls rush headlong into detailed, long-winded narratives, apparently reflecting the way they rush headlong into love itself. If "erotic" means what a girl feels when a boy finally notices her, or when he sweeps her off her feet, or when she is nestled in his arms and dreaming about the future, then adolescent girls can write the book on it.

Notwithstanding these comments, though, girls still voice some troubling thoughts about romantic relationship. In the end, romance also is fraught with complications and maddening realities; girls express being at a loss to contend with the ironies and double standards of gender difference. Frustration abounds at the way love and romance have been constructed for them as girlfriends. As a result, their stories thus contain an undercurrent of powerlessness. Even with romantic love rather than sexuality per se, they ultimately feel trapped; and again, some girls explicitly connect their sense of entrapment to their gender.

That love and romance assume an important place in many teenage girls' lives is fairly easy to discern from their conversations. Girls' ideas about romance are often fairly conventional. As Orenstein reports, they like to think it begins with "candles and flowers." She observed an in-school support group for Latina girls at one of the high schools she visited. One day the leader of the group, Jessica, started talking with the girls about romance.

"How would you like a relationship to be, how do you think about it?"

The girls smile, but they don't answer.

"Do you think that a relationship is about being pressured?"

A few girls shake their heads no.

"No? That's not how you think about it? Because a lot of girls do. How many of you think about it like romance" — Jessica changes her voice to a singsong — "like candles and flowers."

There's giggling assent.[29]

---

29. Orenstein, *SchoolGirls*, 216–17.

"Candles and flowers" are what many adolescent girls prefer to think romance is all about. They readily assent to this construction of the erotic, even while part of them knows that the image is unrealistic or silly. In the abstract, at least, teenage girls often speak cheerfully about the joys of romantic relationship. Thompson reports the following response from a girl she intercepted in a shopping mall:

> Oh, I love romance. I do, I do. I love a lot of things about love.... You know, you get that special feeling. That feels good. I'm going to meet somebody now.... The other ones are just lust, you know. You just like to be with them but this one I love. I know I do.[30]

Despite her relatively lighthearted tone, however, one thing this girl is serious about is the distinction between "love" and "lust," and she claims she can easily tell the difference. She quickly dismisses, moreover, any feelings of lust she may have had for former boyfriends ("the other ones"), as if those feelings were inconsequential because love is "the real thing." She is certain that *this* time she is in love because for her, being in love means having "that special feeling." "That special feeling" defines the erotic for her. She may be so preoccupied with it that she can no longer identify with other erotic feelings she might have once had.

Preoccupation with Romance

Plotting and preparing for romance clearly form among adolescent girls a common preoccupation that can become consuming. For example, one girl admits that dreams about meeting a boy intrude into her other activities:

> If something is going to happen, then I'll daydream. If we're going to have a test or something like that... like if I meet a boy, like what will happen in the future or something....[31]

Some girls even try to be ready for love at any moment, lest it should appear while they are otherwise occupied. Thompson describes her interview with Tracy:

> Tracy started talking about Don the minute we got together. She didn't stop to take off her purple satin jacket. She sat down in the

---

30. Thompson, "Search for Tomorrow," 355.
31. Thompson, "Search for Tomorrow," 361.

middle of a sentence. [Tracy described the day she discovered Don had a crush on her.] Tracy was thrilled. Recently she had bleached her hair and started sleeping in makeup on the expectation that just this kind of romantic encounter might happen at any moment.[32]

When asked to name their hopes and dreams for the future, few teenage girls will *not* mention marriage, or at least romantic relationship. Thompson interviewed one girl just after a relationship of hers had ended unhappily and notes that it was one of the rare times she talked to a girl who seemed to pin her hopes for happiness on something other than romantic love. Even in this instance, however, the girl could not help but include it in her list of dreams:

My idea of what I want to do right now is to get a career that I love, like being a legal secretary or something so that I can be totally independent of a guy. Whereas, if I marry somebody or even live with somebody and they leave me, I won't have anything to worry about because I'll be totally independent. That's definitely what I want to do. There's no question about it. Second of all, I want the ideal relationship with a guy. I guess I want somebody to love me and care about me as much as I do them. I think I deserve that.[33]

All these comments demonstrate that love and romance are resilient themes in girls' everyday discourse. Orenstein noted that concern about love and romance seems an unavoidable part of female adolescence, and she calls this phenomenon "the lure of involvement with boys." She refers to the condition as a "lure" because, despite acknowledging their potential for being hurt and having their reputations damaged, many of the girls she encountered continued to yearn for romantic love.

At Weston [the upper-middle-class school], the girls speak of boys' power to ruin their reputation, to undercut their self-esteem by branding them sluts. Yet, in spite of those hazards, they are still keen to lose themselves in love and are as syrupy as a Harlequin novel in their infatuations.[34]

---

32. Thompson, *Going All the Way,* 17–18.
33. Thompson, "Search for Tomorrow," 356.
34. Orenstein, *SchoolGirls,* 236–37.

Even when girls were more hesitant to become involved with boys because of their fears about sex, Orenstein heard the lure of romance assert
itself. She cites her conversation with Dashelle, a portion of which we
heard above:

> "Girls want boyfriends and all that little mess," [Dashelle] con-
> tinues, "but to me, I think boys distract you from school and
> everything. They can knock things out of your mind. So I don't
> want a boyfriend.... But I don't know. I wish I could talk to you
> in two years when I'm in high school. Maybe I'll have a different
> attitude then; maybe more things come at you in high school and
> maybe you do want a boyfriend, I don't know. I don't know...."[35]

In this case, even Dashelle seems aware of the lure: "maybe you *do* want
a boyfriend."

Romantic relationship often becomes to female adolescents, at least
to an observer, disproportionately important compared to other potential
interests. One indication of this status is the high drama with which girls
describe their encounters with the opposite sex. We can barely imagine a
boy bursting into a researcher's office and breathlessly telling her about
his latest romantic encounter, the way Tracy did with Sharon Thompson.
In addition, the actual episodes girls describe so vividly are often much
briefer and probably much less significant, in the end, than their telling
would have us believe. One of Thompson's earliest and most striking
findings was that girls' narrative ability about romance is extremely well
developed. Thompson explains:

> These stories had a polished quality, and I think this was because
> they were rehearsed. These were the stories that teenage girls spend
> hundreds of hours telling each other, going over and over detail and
> possibility as part of the process of constructing and reconstructing
> sexual and existential meaning for themselves.[36]

A polished ability to tell stories may simply mean that girls have learned
to imitate the discourse about sex and romance to which they are so
routinely exposed. The romantic tale (teen magazines, soap operas, talk
shows, and so on) is ubiquitous in their lives and is a powerful teacher.

---

35. Orenstein, *SchoolGirls*, 237–38.
36. Thompson, "Search for Tomorrow," 351.

But one might also argue that romance is genuinely exciting to them and that it captivates them. Romance may be "erotic" for many adolescent girls in the sense of driving their energies and passions. As Thompson puts it, "sex and romance are the organizing principles, the fundamental projects in many, many teenage girls' lives."[37]

Arguably, that romance is erotic — or, to put it another way, that Eros is reduced to romance — may be unfortunate and at times unhealthy. When girls interpret and even measure their own lives against romantic fairy tales, something seems backward. Adolescent girls appear to be investing their own particular lives with trite meanings, as though girls really believe in the premise of the Sleeping Beauty tale: that their *raison d'être* is to wait for the right man who will make them fall in love and give them happiness ever after. They seem to share Sleeping Beauty's own expectation — that fate dictates finding the handsome prince, falling in love, and ultimately marrying — and they accept this pattern as the female "quest."

> Romance is the quest for sexual destiny, the search for a partner custom-made by the stars, the genes, or by so many random, subtle, and exquisitely specific factors that the process may as well be ascribed to magic. It is the search for the one or the ones who will recognize and validate by loving or having sex with the seeker, the one waiting to be found.[38]

Nevertheless, however unhealthy this outlook may be, girls' erotic passion for romance is not false or perverted. It is real. To deny that the meaning of Eros for many adolescent girls *is* a genuine passion for romantic relationship is difficult. Their desire to have a boyfriend is what they would identify as "erotic," were they to use that language.

A love-struck teen's desire for romance is not disingenuous, nor is it simply masquerading as other desires. Rather, the desire to have a boyfriend *is* the erotic desire, but constructing the erotic as romantic involvement is not without problems. Any construction of the erotic is problematic insofar as it constricts the range of passions a person is free to feel. If a girl believes that receiving attention and being swept off her feet is a thrill, she will tend to reconstruct in this fashion even the most banal romantic encounters. This approach, however, can twist the reality

---

37. Thompson, "Search for Tomorrow," 354.
38. Thompson, "Search for Tomorrow," 354. Thompson describes romance in fairy tale terms because they reflect the way girls think about it.

of erotic situations out of proportion. For example, when asked to recall her feelings about a sexual experience (which happened to be with another girl), a young college student in effect admitted to Thompson that she could remember more about what she thought she should feel than what she actually felt.

How did you feel about [the sexual experience]?

Pretty adventurous . . . I was very conscious of the romantic or that I was supposed to feel swept away. I really didn't have a clue of what I was supposed to have been doing, but I was very conscious of what I was supposed to have been feeling and sort of felt that way. Looking back, I don't think that was necessarily true arousal, but it was perceived to be.[39]

This young woman had "read hundreds of Harlequin and other heterosexual romance novels,"[40] and therefore she knew what she was supposed to feel: "swept away." She is not entirely clear, looking back, about what her feelings actually were at the time — she only "sort of felt" swept away and, in retrospect, she is not at all sure she was aroused — but she does have a clear sense of what she *expected* her feelings to be. She admits that she perceived herself to be aroused at the time because she thought she was "supposed to" feel that way. That this narrator is a lesbian does not apparently change her internalization of stereotypical constructions of sexual desire.[41]

These stereotypes genuinely excite many adolescent girls. After all, stereotypes persist for a reason. If they had no appeal, they would lose their meaning and significance. In fact, even girls who may not be enthralled by romantic love feel they should present themselves as enthralled by it, so powerful is the idea. If falling in love is the ultimate goal, then presumably a girl should be triumphant when she has succeeded in reaching this goal. One girl who deliberately rejected serious romantic and

---

39. Thompson, "Search for Tomorrow," 366.
40. Thompson, "Search for Tomorrow," 366.
41. In other words, this information contradicts assumptions made by some feminist theologians of the erotic (and some feminist theorists) that being a lesbian "liberates" a woman from cultural constructions of femininity. On the contrary, I would argue that same-sex desire probably tends to be harder for girls to reconcile with perceived expectations about desire. Although such research is beyond the scope of this project, much anecdotal evidence suggests that same-sex desire and perceived expectations about desire can be very confusing for adolescents.

sexual involvement astutely observed that other girls' claims of true love seemed to her like "keeping up a front":

> I think it's a lot of fronts. The girls I know that are in serious re-lationships . . . when they're around everybody else they have to act like they're in love and you can tell that they're not. And they talk about "Oh, I'm so in love, I'm so in love," twenty-four hours a day, and you know that if they really felt that way, they wouldn't have to keep dwelling on the subject.[42]

But harm can result in letting the romantic quest enthrall oneself. Con-structing the erotic around romance tends to fuel obsession. When romance becomes so central to a girl's life that she thinks about it "twenty-four hours a day," she risks losing interest in and commitment to other things such as school, friendship, and sports. She may jeopardize other re-lationships and put other projects on hold in her exclusive focus on finding and keeping a boyfriend.

Vulnerability to Loss and Emptiness

Some girls appear to realize that the erotic is highly constructed and reg-ister some awareness of their discomfort with that realization. Often this realization becomes most clear after a romantic relationship ends and they see the romance for its true worth to them. Many girls reported to Thomp-son, for example, that after finally overcoming the feelings attendant to a romantic breakup, they realized how obsessed with the relationship they had become and how they then rued their own memories. One girl's description of her obsession is quite vivid:

> I wrote songs and poems about him all the time. I was obsessed with him. One time, believe it or not, after he'd been at our house and was drinking coffee with Tony and my dad, I put his coffee cup in my room on my shelf and I drank out of it after he did.[43]

Another girl talked about her distress in terms of realizing that, through the relationship and its loss, she had turned into an utterly different person:

---

42. Thompson, *Going All the Way*, 65.
43. Thompson, *Going All the Way*, 40.

I've become very quiet. That is not me . . . I didn't stop living. . . . But
I am not the same person. I'm very inactive. I'm eating a lot. I'm
gaining weight because of him. But that's only little parts of it. I
can't even begin to explain how I feel inside.[44]

An undertone of disquiet and even disgust is present in these narratives.
The first girl sounds incredulous remembering how she saved her boyfriend's coffee cup. The second girl expresses discomfort and even dismay
over letting herself change so much, just because of a boy — "I'm gaining
weight because of him." Apparently, in reevaluating the importance of
romance to them, they were seeing themselves anew. Perhaps they were
even beginning to revisit their assumptions about what being a girl and
what being in a romantic relationship mean.

Thompson takes pains to point out that female adolescent angst over
failed love affairs should not be read as self-indulgent melodrama. Investing so much emotional energy in a relationship with someone — and,
more importantly, staking one's identity and worth upon being in relationship — would leave anyone vulnerable to feelings of loss and emptiness.
Genuine anguish follows upon placing something at the center of one's
life and then losing it. This anguish, Thompson reports, is exacerbated if a
girl has had sex with her boyfriend. As she notes, the double standard for
sexual intercourse still means that sex carries greater consequences for a
girl than for a boy; she risks more in self-esteem, reputation, and identity
than he does if she consents to "going all the way." Consider the distress
captured in the following poem, which Thompson reports almost all the
girls in one town she visited had copied down:

> When I met you, I liked you.
> When I liked you, I loved you.
> When I loved you, I let you.
> When I let you, I lost you.[45]

How do teenage girls make sense of their own confusion, obsession,
and discomfort with respect to sex and romance? How do they interpret
what is happening to them? As one might expect, girls have different levels
of insight into their preoccupations and obsessions. Many girls seem to
be aware, however, of the role that gender plays in their experience. As

---

44. Thompson, *Going All the Way,* 40.
45. Thompson, *Going All the Way,* 27.

I have pointed out already, they are usually keenly aware that boys rarely suffer the way they do.

The Need for Structural Change

Girls' experiences of the erotic are clearly not all the same. Their narratives reveal significant differences. Yet, even more striking differences are apparent between the girls quoted in this chapter and the type of woman conjured up by Audre Lorde and other feminist theologians of the erotic. The narrators we have heard scarcely sound like they are discovering their "lifeforce." Therefore, to express great optimism at this point about female adolescent sexuality is inappropriate. The cumulative distress of perplexity, confusion, self-doubt, and obsession voiced in these narratives borders on the tragic. The researchers who listened to scores of adolescent girls in the course of their work all expressed dismay at their findings. Looking retrospectively at her work, Sharon Thompson writes, "The pain, fear, and disappointment that most girls reported especially in the early years of this study were hurtful in and of themselves. They not only decreased the probability of effective contraceptive practice. They undercut girls' sense of well-being and hope and generated depression and amnesia."[46] Researchers concluded their work with less rather than more faith in girls' power to change their own circumstances.

For adolescent girls simply to muster up more confidence and courage from within themselves will not suffice. Their conflicts run too deeply. The "any woman can" motto of voluntarism, as Sandra Bartky calls it, rings hollow in the face of the skepticism and despair we have heard. In other words, even if teenage girls reach deeply within themselves, they will not necessarily tap into a source of wisdom and strength that can empower them.

On the other hand, one cannot conclude from the evidence that teenage girls who voice distress about the erotic, or preoccupation with one particularly narrow form of it, are duped or misinformed. The girls we have heard seem more astute, even about their own problems, than this assessment would suggest. They are often the first to realize the harm in their choices. They are troubled by being troubled, and while one could argue

---

46. Thompson, "Search for Tomorrow," 350.

that this feeling represents the first step in enlightenment, perhaps, too, insofar as troubles persist, enlightenment is an insufficient remedy.

After listening to the voices of these adolescent girls, therefore, we have no particular reason to conclude that the erotic as such will be a reliably liberating force for them. On the other hand, neither should we conclude that the erotic is inherently bad, or that teenage girls inevitably suffer from it. None of the researchers drawn upon in this chapter concludes that the difficulty reconciling Eros and femaleness is a foregone conclusion; all of these researchers believe this difficulty to be a political problem, not a biological or "natural" one.

In other words, the resolution to problems in erotic experience requires a structural rather than an individual approach. If structural conditions were changed, individuals would still have their own particular personalities, experiences, and problems and might not escape all the dilemmas of desire. But those dilemmas would take different shape in a different social context. In particular, if gender equality were fully realized, whatever dilemmas and despair still characterized human sexuality would not be so closely linked to gender. Problems with eroticism would still arise, but they would presumably arise equally for boys and girls. Therefore, feminist theologians and ethicists need to be more suspicious about the structural relationships between gender inequality and the erotic. The continued attraction for so many girls, for example, of conventional romantic roles warrants investigation. Why and how are girls lured into relishing romantic relationship the way they do? The answers to these and other questions will never come from looking at girls *qua* individuals; rather, they call for a shift in perspective toward the structural conditions of girls' lives.

Finally, these stories suggest that girls scarcely need more advocacy regarding relationality. We cannot conclude from this evidence that for their erotic flourishing, the closer the relational bonding the better. These girls seem to need some relief from their self-imposed burden of finding and sustaining intimate relationships (at least romantic ones). If the erotic is so closely associated with relationality as feminist theologians of the erotic have suggested, this association only reinforces adolescent girls' tendency toward it. Building a moral discourse about erotic love or sexual activity that overemphasizes the values of being in relationship potentially sends the wrong message to this particular group.

In short, if we were to listen only to feminist theologians of the erotic about sexual ethics, we would gain the wrong impression of sexuality. Adolescents' experiences generally do not fit their mold. Adolescents' problems do not fit their diagnoses. Consequently, what adolescents need rather than more feminist theology of the erotic is a more practical sexual ethic. The rest of this book moves in that direction. In the next chapter, I use the work of psychologists and psychoanalytic theorists to deepen our understanding of the dilemmas adolescent girls face with respect to Eros. The study then concludes with a proposal for developing a sexual ethic based upon trust.

FIVE

Understanding the Construction
of the Erotic

> But no matter whether my probings made me happier or sadder, I kept on
> probing to know.   — Zora Neale Hurston, *Dust Tracks on a Road*

L ISTENING TO THE VOICES of the girls in chapter 4 can be frustrating. Perhaps believing that erotic relationships are really as bad as
these girls make them sound can be difficult. One might be tempted to
conclude that girls as distressed as these simply need to assert themselves
more vigorously, ignore the distorted messages of mainstream culture,
and learn to speak up for themselves. One might interpret their primary
problem as one of confidence and the corresponding solution as one of
developing some assertive skills. In terms of girls' overblown and dispro-
portionate desires for romance, one might be inclined to counsel them
simply to control their emotions and to want something besides a boyfriend. "Just don't be so concerned about boys. Cultivate friendships, get
involved in other activities, develop other interests." This advice is heard
on many a talk show, printed in countless teen magazine columns, and
doled out everywhere by parents, older siblings, and friends.

From a feminist and theological perspective as well, hearing so much
apathy and anxiety voiced about the erotic can be frustrating. Like one
feminist theorist, we may discover that "[a]t times we are shocked by
how much the reality of woman's condition differs from what we, in our
minds, have long since determined it should be."[1] If a feminist theologian
or ethicist has long since determined that men and women alike should enjoy erotic experiences as part of God's good creation, learning that erotic
conditions are often so dismal for girls in the younger generation can be

---

1. Jessica Benjamin, *Bonds of Love: Psychoanalysis, Feminism, and the Problem of Domination*
(New York: Pantheon Books, 1988), 87.

shocking. Their stories present a challenge to contemporary theologies because they throw into doubt the confidence in the erotic that characterizes much theological discourse. If a feminist theologian of the erotic were to give advice to the girls in chapter 4, or offer an interpretation of their stories, how might it go? With less emphasis than heard from mothers and magazine columnists on controlling or redirecting emotions, and more emphasis on accepting and celebrating them, the advice might run something like this: "You should not feel ashamed of your erotic feelings. Everyone has them; they are a gift from God. Pay attention to them. They can put you in touch with some of the most important things in life. Sexuality is wonderful. It embodies, after all, the love two people have for one another. Nonsexual erotic experiences are also wonderful. So if you would only trust the erotic feelings buried inside you, you would discover true fulfillment." In a more theoretical vein, feminist theologians of the erotic might interpret adolescent narratives as evidence of the oppressive social structures and religious doctrines that keep female eroticism repressed and docile.

Advising teenage girls to be more confident and assertive, and to develop other interests, is too little advice too late. Such an approach casts girls' behaviors as "problems" needing solving rather than as symptoms of deeper problems regarding sex, gender, culture, and power. Moreover, as we have already seen, advice about asserting themselves contradicts many girls' experience that when they *are* assertive, they risk others' ridicule and rejection. Being told to divert their passion away from romance likewise contradicts what they have heard for years — that romance is every girl's dream and that their destiny lies in finding a man, settling down, and living happily ever after. While genuine concern for girls' plight may motivate the type of advice that teen magazine columnists, talk show hosts, and anxious mothers offer, such advice conveys naiveté about the gender politics that both give rise to and reinforce that plight.

But so, too, is the advice from feminist theologies of the erotic naive. In some ways, their celebration of the goodness of sexuality and the erotic might inspire those girls who know that they want to express their desires. But these theologies inadequately address girls whose self-doubt, confusion, and obsession entrap them.

This chapter, therefore, turns instead to an interpretation offered in psychological and psychoanalytic theories about how the erotic is constructed for and by adolescent girls. While not claiming that one can universalize girls' experience across cultures or even in contemporary U.S. society, the similarity of experience in at least a significant number of girls' accounts, as shown in the previous chapter, warrants a theoretical inquiry into female adolescent Eros. In particular, participant-observers write of being arrested by the repeated protestations of ignorance they heard from the girls they interviewed. Girls routinely qualified their statements about the erotic with confessions of not knowing: "I don't like to think . . ."; "I don't know how to bring up the subject"; "Do you know what I mean? I'm not sure I do, myself!"; "I don't know"; "I just wish I could forget it"; "I don't know." This uncertainty could simply characterize the way teenagers talk today, were it not for the fact that such disclaimers also too often prefaced much conflict. Given the multiple and often contradictory ideas about the erotic they have to reconcile, no wonder teenage girls express some confusion. Surely we can't expect *them* to resolve the meaning of adolescent sexuality! But this need for reconciliation does not necessarily explain why they frequently seem unsure of what they themselves know. Why can't girls figure out what to say when asked to share their own thoughts and feelings? Our three also note that when girls talked about erotic or romantic relationship, consistent claims of optimism preceded equally consistent expressions of disappointment. This contradiction indicates yet another puzzle to solve: Why are girls still preoccupied with being in relationship despite gnawing doubts about its value?

In this chapter I seek to shed light on these questions by studying the peculiar developmental hurdles young girls in American culture face in acquiring a sense of self and learning how to be in relationship. (The two, as we shall see, are interrelated.) The chapter argues that the conflicts and contradictions heard in girls' discourse about the erotic stem from their difficulty negotiating those developmental hurdles. By learning what typically happens to undermine the smooth process of self-development in girls from early childhood to adolescence, we are able to shed more light on their strange obliqueness, once they reach adolescence, regarding Eros. By learning what typically happens to exacerbate preoccupation with relational issues, we can also begin to understand girls' puzzling obsession over romantic relationship.

As theoreticians across disciplines agree, during adolescence girls' powers of reasoning (not intelligence) about many things does indeed appear to become stifled. At some point in adolescence, many girls begin to claim ambivalence, perplexity, and conflict about the same issues they had felt sure about when they were eight or nine or ten. Generations of psychologists and psychoanalysts have noted this phenomenon, but with no consensus about its cause.[2] Theoreticians also observe that adolescence often ushers in an intense interest in interpersonal relationship; many observers have long simply assumed that adolescent girls naturally take an interest in romance. Today, feminist psychologists, psychoanalysts, developmental theorists, and object relations theorists are raising doubts about traditional theories of female adolescence and are studying these issues anew. Their interpretations are proving illuminating and persuasive. These theorists include Carol Gilligan and her colleagues, who have attended closely to issues of "voice" and gender in the psychological and moral development of preadolescent and adolescent girls as well as women; Lori Stern, a Gilligan protegée who brings psychoanalytic theory to the techniques of the Gilligan school; and Jessica Benjamin and Nancy Chodorow, two neo-Freudians who employ object relations theory to study the interrelationships of gender, sexuality, family, power, and culture.

Briefly, the theory I develop on the basis of these studies goes as follows: Girls' conflict and ambivalence around the erotic may actually be an expression of a more profound developmental conflict, one introduced in infancy, solidified in early childhood, and revisited again during adolescence. A psychic conflict arises between separation and attachment, experienced by boys but exacerbated in girls whose gender in this culture is a handicap in attempting to overcome it. The conflict can also be described as a paradox between yearning for individuality and yearning for connection with others. While not solely responsible, this paradox, and the strategies girls mount to resolve it, contributes to the ambiguity, perplexity, and conflict we hear dominating girls' discourse about the erotic. At the same time, this paradox also helps to explain why adolescent girls can at times appear so certain about their desire to be involved with boys

---

2. Psychoanalytic theorists and clinicians from Freud on have accepted girls' "regressive" phase as a normal part of the pattern of female adolescent development, and they have explained it in terms of penis envy and the castration complex. See Sigmund Freud, "The Transformation of Puberty," in *Three Essays on the Theory of Sexuality* (New York: Basic Books, 1905/1962); Karen Horney, "The Flight from Womanhood," *International Journal of Psychoanalysis* 7 (1926); Helene Deutsch, *Psychology of Women,* vol. 1 (New York: Grune & Stratton, 1944); Clara Thompson, *Interpersonal Psychoanalysis* (New York: Basic Books, 1964). Recently, however, feminist psychoanalytic theorists have begun challenging these traditional explanations — and challenging as well the "normalcy" of a regression to passivity. I discuss their work in this chapter.

and so magnetized by romance. At a psychic level, they choose relationship over self and become "sure" that they desire love and romance above all. Structured into adolescent girls' conscious ideas about the erotic, in other words, are unconscious ideas about what being a girl means and what it takes to be in relationship with others.

Developmental Theory

The work of Carol Gilligan and her colleagues in the Harvard Project on Women's Psychology and Girls' Development provides a valuable way to interpret the struggles that female adolescents face. Gilligan's group has studied girls' development during preadolescence and adolescence by interviewing girls and then analyzing the speech patterns that recur in the interview transcripts — for example, the number of times a girl says "I don't know" in her responses to questions. Using this methodology, they document and interpret the stifling of reasoning that typically occurs in female adolescence. The work of the Gilligan school suggests an explanation for this problem that links it to gender inequality: Girls' reasoning becomes stifled because at this particular point in development they are attempting simultaneously to claim their own voice and to modulate it to conform to constructions of femaleness.

Brown and Gilligan and "Approaching the Wall"

The early work of the Gilligan school attempted to show that women speak in a "different voice" from men — a voice that makes more frequent reference to relationship and the moral interconnection of persons.[3] Gilligan and her colleagues then began to trace this difference back through successively earlier stages in female development, eventually all the way back to girlhood and preadolescence. In addition to interviewing younger subjects, they also began to characterize the phenomenon they were study-

---

3. See especially Carol Gilligan, *In a Different Voice: Psychological Theory and Women's Development* (Cambridge: Harvard University Press, 1982). Feminists have highly lauded and highly criticized this text. Some interpreters of Gilligan's work criticize her for positing essential differences between women and men; others charge that she insufficiently critiques the social and political structures of gender that generate the differences she notes. My own view is that Gilligan's work has changed and developed over time (perhaps to take some of these criticisms into account), and that her later work is more nuanced with respect to the relationship between gender difference and gender inequality than was *In a Different Voice*. While I still disagree with some of what Gilligan says, I think ethicists and others ought to pay more attention to her later work; references to Gilligan in the literature still tend to be references to *In a Different Voice*.

ing in terms of a "crisis" rather than a difference, suggesting that attention to relationship and interconnection may not simply be a natural characteristic of women's reasoning, but rather a strategy for coping with the structural conditions of their lives as women (and in particular, as caregivers). This revised thesis guides *Meeting at the Crossroads,* published in 1992 by Lyn Mikel Brown and Carol Gilligan. In this book, Brown and Gilligan present the results of their 1986–90 study of girls attending the Laurel School, a private day school for girls in Cleveland.[4] Throughout this study, Gilligan's group of researchers was particularly intent on analyzing girls' loss of voice over the course of preadolescent and adolescent development. They strove to detail and clarify how and why female discourse is muted upon entry into adolescence, and even further strained as adolescence progresses; and they concluded that "[w]omen, in contrast [to men], tended to speak of themselves as living in connection with others and yet described a relational crisis: a giving up of voice, an abandonment of self, for the sake of becoming a good woman and having relationships."[5]

Through the process of interview and analysis, Brown and Gilligan discovered that starting at roughly age ten or eleven, many girls' discourse changed significantly when talking about interpersonal matters such as friendship, family, and moral decisions. Girls appeared to become dissociated from their own powers of reasoning and discernment. (Dissociation is not necessarily the same thing as abandonment. Girls still have the ability to reason, Brown and Gilligan argue, but choose to relinquish it.) When they were only a couple of years younger, they did not hesitate to state the differences they discerned in people's moral character by saying, for example, that they approved of certain people's actions and disapproved of others'. But at some point during preadolescence, many of the girls appeared to develop a palpable fear of voicing anything that would force them into claiming a distinct opinion. Some girls said they feared even the appearance of giving priority to themselves over others and the consequent loss of friendship. For instance, they would reserve their criticism of a friend's bad behavior so as to preserve the friendship and their own

4. Most girls who attended the Laurel School were from middle-class or upper-middle-class homes, but 20 percent were from working-class homes. Fourteen percent were girls of color, and 86 percent were white.

5. Lyn Mikel Brown and Carol Gilligan, *Meeting at the Crossroads: Women's Psychology and Girls' Development* (Cambridge: Harvard University Press, 1992), 2.

"niceness." Some said that risking their status as a nice and friendly person by voicing any negative opinion of a popular girl in school would be treacherous. Others said that learning to be less outspoken was simply easier. On the home front, girls refused to attribute to themselves feelings of outrage at unfair parental rules, even though other comments clearly indicated their anger.[6]

In many cases, these preteens still knew what they thought, or believed they did, but intentionally withheld their opinions. A ten-year-old girl named Noura admitted to her interviewer that she had *learned* how to say "I don't know" to avoid disagreement. She reported several instances when she would deliberately equivocate, saying "sometimes, but not always," when asked for some judgment on an interpersonal matter. She described how she would always attempt to go along with her friends, even if such an action meant disavowing thoughts and opinions she held that went contrary to theirs.[7] Brown and Gilligan write, "The two worst things Noura's friends can accuse her of, it seems, are either not knowing and saying the wrong things or knowing and saying the wrong things."[8] Many girls were less self-aware than Noura of what they were doing, but nevertheless reported no longer being able to make up their minds. In interviews, they questioned aloud the judgments they had just made to the interviewer. When presented with hypothetical problems, such as an argument between two friends or a conflict among demands on their time, they simply refused to discern any solutions.

If Brown and Gilligan found girls having difficulty figuring out what to say about hypothetical dilemmas, we can only imagine girls' difficulty with actual conflicts about their femininity in a culture where the threat of "becoming a slut" constantly looms. Brown and Gilligan found that older girls (those in adolescence) not only tended to withhold their responses to situations, but also questioned more frequently the certainty of the responses they had formulated. As girls became older, they more frequently prefaced statements of opinion and judgment with disclaimers such as "I'm not sure, but..." and to qualify their statements with phrases such as "I mean" and "I don't know."[9] They began to contradict themselves

6. Brown and Gilligan, *Meeting at the Crossroads,* especially 89–106.
7. Brown and Gilligan, *Meeting at the Crossroads,* 112–13.
8. Brown and Gilligan, *Meeting at the Crossroads,* 112.
9. Brown and Gilligan, *Meeting at the Crossroads,* 133. In analyzing speech patterns, Brown and Gilligan call "I don't know" the "bellwether of dissociation" and "I mean" "a sign of the

more frequently and to disavow in one sentence what they had just said in the previous one. For example, when Judy was asked to explain what might resolve some severe tension at home between her siblings, father, and stepmother, Judy struggled even to say anything definite:

> I don't know, because I don't — I don't know. I mean, I do know. I just like — I can't explain it. I don't know what, how to put it into words.

> *What does it feel like? or what does it look like?*

> I don't know, it's just like if — I don't know, it's like, I don't know, I can't even begin to explain it, because I don't even know if I know what it is. So I can't really explain it. Because I don't know. I don't even know like in my brain or in my heart, what I am really feeling. I mean I don't know if it's pain or upsetness or sad — I don't know.[10]

Some girls even started to express fear about their own thoughts. At age thirteen, Noura became apprehensive over the mere prospect of having to think. In answer to an interview question about her response to a troubling situation among her friends, she said, "Sometimes I think it's just too confusing to think about, and I shouldn't really. . . . Sometimes I'm afraid to think one way. . . . I try to keep myself from thinking that I dislike it."[11] Brown and Gilligan note with disappointment and irony that even though the older girls they interviewed had keener minds with which they might access solutions to problems, they nevertheless spoke more tentatively, and appeared even more perplexed, than younger girls. They write: "The slipperiness of words and the treachery of relationships which ten- and eleven-year-old girls are acutely aware of have become solidified and normalized by twelve and thirteen."[12]

The similarities between the discourse of Laurel School girls and the girls in chapter 4 are striking. Just as girls seem to dissociate themselves from their own thoughts about the erotic, they seem to dissociate themselves from their thoughts and feelings more generally. Just as girls' ability

---

struggle to connect herself with knowing, her mind with relationship." One girl said "I don't know" six times more often in her eighth-grade interview than in her sixth-grade one, and "I mean" twice as often (p. 133).

10. Brown and Gilligan, *Meeting at the Crossroads,* 135.
11. Brown and Gilligan, *Meeting at the Crossroads,* 122.
12. Brown and Gilligan, *Meeting at the Crossroads,* 169.

to make good decisions about sexuality appears hampered, so, too, their reasoning about friendships and family relationships appears weakened.

Brown and Gilligan named the phenomenon they detected in female adolescent discourse "approaching the wall," for when they analyzed the patterns in the interview transcripts, they felt as though they were watching girls confront some insurmountable obstacle blocking their emotional and intellectual progress. The gradual loss of voice among female adolescents that they detected does not represent, they argue, a retardation in girls' development, as plausible as this might seem. Rather, this loss represents a way of battling against an obstacle, an active response to a particularly difficult dilemma. The "wall" that adolescent girls approach is the paradox of self-assertion versus connection to others, which represents a seeming contradiction because girls do not know how to stay true to themselves and simultaneously loyal to others. The two appear mutually exclusive. In response to this dilemma, girls literally silence themselves when faced with situations that seemingly force them to choose. Granted, the strategy may not ultimately succeed, but that girls try at all to circumvent "the wall" and continue to grow as individuals, according to these researchers, is impressive. Girls' self-silencing, in other words, should be viewed with sympathy rather than exasperation.

In *Meeting at the Crossroads,* Brown and Gilligan offer several reasons that "the wall" materializes during adolescence (rather than earlier or later in life). They suggest that as girls reach adolescence, they have better cognitive skills with which to "decode" the messages they have received about gender, sexuality, love, and morality.[13] They begin to realize that "scripts" pervade discourses on these topics, and they are able to place themselves as actors within the scripts. At the same time, however, they are not yet able to deconstruct the scripts and hence they remain actors — doomed to repeat their lines rather than invent new ones — which creates a profound and painful disjuncture between acting a part and realizing it *is* a part.

Supporting this theory, one fourteen-year-old girl named Victoria mocked the gamelike nature of romance with a clarity of insight beyond her years:

> [Relationships are] like a little game you play. You know, you don't really care, and you sit there and say "I love you," and if they say

13. See especially 159–62.

they love you back, you know that means they want to go farther the next time they see you or whatever. . . . Yah, it's a game. I mean it's like preparing you for the ultimate game which is like marriage, you know. The trick.[14]

In the face of such a disjuncture, Brown and Gilligan argue that one understandable response is to relinquish one's voice (if one does not become cynical, as this girl seems to have become). What has seemed true, after all, has in some sense been unmasked as false, and yet alternative ways of thinking and acting do not yet appear possible. If no one around you confirms your sense that romance is largely a construct rather than a natural end, and that the myth of true love is just that, for example, then you might very well begin to doubt your own ability to understand and form your own thoughts about these things. Perplexity and uncertainty characterize girls' responses. Brown and Gilligan write:

Judy, Noura, and Victoria, culturally inscribed and socially ͻnalized notions of womanhood which specify the normal, al, the desirable, the good, and the bad woman, enter girls' tions and a struggle breaks out — a struggle to know what ͻw, to rely on their feelings, to hold onto their experiences r relationships as a way of grounding themselves. Asked if ever been in a situation where what she knows to be true ͺperience is different from what others are saying and doing, Anna replies, "All the time . . . that's my life."[15]

Brown and Gilligan also suggest that when adolescent girls do speak up against the ironies and hypocrisies that they are beginning to notice, people who do not want to hear what they have to say frequently tell them to be quiet. Consequently, they gradually jettison their attempts to challenge what they hear and choose silence instead. Brown and Gilligan dub this phenomenon "the tyranny of nice and kind."[16] A girl who points out the irony of adult behavior is considered "not nice." From an early age, too, girls are told that disagreeing with friends or adults is not "nice" because it might create conflict and hurt feelings. Girls come to understand

14. Brown and Gilligan, *Meeting at the Crossroads,* 153.
15. Brown and Gilligan, *Meeting at the Crossroads,* 166.
16. See especially 53–62.

the implicit threat that if they are critical of others, people will leave or ignore them; in other words, they will suffer a loss of relationship. The imperative to be nice and kind tyrannizes their sense of self. They grow increasingly silent, forget how to formulate opinions, and relinquish their entitlement to ideas and passions.

In summary, Brown and Gilligan argue that girls both know and yet do not know what they are doing when they mute their own voices. On the one hand, they are astute enough to know that silence is strategically useful for them, and yet on the other hand, they are not experienced enough to realize that they run the risk of genuinely dissociating from their own thoughts and feelings.

> Girls at the edge of adolescence face a central relational crisis: to speak what they know through experience of themselves and of relationships causes political problems — disagreement with authorities, disrupting relationships — while not to speak leaves a residue of psychological problems: false relationships and confusion as to what they think and feel.[17]

Brown and Gilligan's findings are important to our discussion of the erotic because they confirm that the erotic, like most areas of personal expression and interpersonal negotiation, is a site of conflict, if not crisis. In other words, that girls and women are repressed or unenlightened about their erotic selves is simply not the case. The situation is even more disturbing: Girls and women sense the hidden costs of failing to flourish erotically and yet do not know how to avoid paying them. They are not so much duped or brainwashed by sexism as they are actively engaged in a struggle to construct a sense of self despite it, a struggle that often ironically manifests itself in hampered moral agency. Their silence may not be eloquent, but it bespeaks a complex problem. Frequently, girls themselves sense a problem and express frustration at their own impotence to overcome it. They are all too aware of what theologians must remember — maintaining a meaningful sense of self as a female and at the same time maintaining without contradiction meaningful erotic relationships with others is no easy task.

---

17. Brown and Gilligan, *Meeting at the Crossroads,* 214.

Stern and "Disavowing the Self"

Psychotherapist and educator Lori Stern, a Gilligan protegée, has further studied the puzzling phenomenon of "knowing yet not knowing" that Gilligan and her colleagues identified. While Gilligan is not unsympathetic to psychoanalytic theory, her work does not explore the psychodynamics of "approaching the wall," so we must turn elsewhere. Concurring with Brown and Gilligan that girls face pressures to forget or deny their own desires and thoughts, Stern thought that girls' self-silencing as a response merited further investigation. She gave a name to the phenomenon — "disavowing the self" — and strove to explain it. To Stern, the phenomenon first appeared as a "startling retrenchment" in female development because girls who had previously been very forthright and confident seemed to change significantly.[18] By "disavowing the self," Stern means the way that "some girls, who in pre-adolescence demonstrate a solid sense of self, begin in adolescence to renounce and devalue their perceptions, beliefs, thoughts, and feelings."[19]

As Stern notes, generations of psychologists and psychoanalysts have observed this same phenomenon, but with no definite consensus about its cause. Freud wrote about how girls enter a "regressive" phase in which they become less assertive, question their own feelings and decisions, and generally lose their previously firm sense of self. Freud accepted this phase as part of the normal pattern of female development and justified the regression by saying that girls were suddenly expressing their repressed envy of the male penis.[20] In 1926, Karen Horney dubbed this phase "the flight from womanhood" because she thought that during the oedipal phase girls were rejecting their femininity. Horney sought an explanation in the differences between girls' and boys' genitalia, and yet she also acknowledged the importance of culture and society:

> It seems to me impossible to judge to how great a degree the unconscious motives for the flight from womanhood are reinforced by the actual social subordination of women. One might conceive of the connection as an interaction of psychic and social factors.[21]

---

18. Lori Stern, "Disavowing the Self in Female Adolescence," *Women and Therapy* 2, no. 3–4 (1991): 105.

19. Stern, "Disavowing the Self," 105.

20. Sigmund Freud, "The Transformation of Puberty," in *Three Essays on the Theory of Sexuality* (New York: Basic Books, 1905/1962).

21. Karen Horney, "The Flight from Womanhood: The Masculinity Complex in Women as Viewed by Men and Women," *International Journal of Psychoanalysis* 7 (1926): 338.

In 1942, Clara Thompson dismissed the idea that women's regression and feelings of inferiority were purely biological, as Freud had postulated, and sought to interpret clinical observations of women's resistance to femininity as cultural and political resistance:

> However, there are other implications in the idea of accepting the feminine rôle — it may include the acceptance of the whole group of attitudes considered feminine by the culture at the time. In such a sense acceptance of the feminine rôle may not be an affirmative attitude at all but an expression of submission and resignation. It may mean choosing the path of least resistance with the sacrifice of important parts of the self for security.[22]

In 1944, Helene Deutsch continued the investigation, acknowledging that an increase in passivity inaugurates a young woman's development.[23]

While each of these theorists were significantly reinterpreting Freud, they continued to present girls' self-devaluation, silencing, and renunciation as "normal" features of the transition into adolescence, according to Stern. Stern argued that these behaviors were not normal and warranted further analysis. Like Brown and Gilligan, Stern believed disavowal of self to be more of a crisis requiring special explanation than a natural part of female development and therefore decided that psychoanalytic theories needed still more feminist interpretation.

Stern argues that disavowing the self is a sophisticated and even creative attempt to circumvent the dilemma between choosing self and choosing others that adolescence brings. She posits that girls begin to anticipate a loss of self and that they struggle, even creatively, to prevent it. When they disavow their judgments and feelings, they do so in hopes of retaining them privately while keeping them from others, according to Stern. Although ultimately to retain one's feelings while simultaneously forfeiting the verbal expression of them may be impossible, girls attempt this strategy anyway because it keeps them from affecting adversely any of their relationships.

Stern quotes Sheila, a girl she interviewed once a year for three years. During the first interview, Sheila had confidently described herself in the following way: "I live by my rules because I don't look at what other

---

22. Clara Thompson, "Cultural Pressures in the Psychology of Women," *Psychiatry* 5, no. 3 (August 1942): 338.
23. Helene Deutsch, *Psychology of Women*, vol. 1 (New York: Grune & Stratton, 1944).

people do. I look at what is best for me."[24] Two years later, however, she expressed quite a different attitude:

> There is always that little part jumping up in the back saying hey me, hey me, you are not worthwhile.

And why not?

> Because people have shown it. Because my relationships have proven that.

How can they show that? How do other people know?

> Other people say it has to be true because you are stupid, you don't know it yourself, you are not even worthwhile to know the truth. Other people must know it.

Do you believe that?

> In a way.

And in another way?

> In another way, I think I must be smarter because I haven't let them in.[25]

Sheila both concurs and does not concur with other people's opinion of her as "stupid" and "not worthwhile." She knows and trusts herself privately but disavows herself publicly to others. She can maintain this paradoxical stance because she doesn't "let others in." They do not need to know what she thinks, and she believes this strategy is "smart."

Even though such a strategy is ultimately doomed, because the dissonance between positive and negative self-evaluations is too unstable, disavowing the self *is* "smart" — a subtle and creative response to a particular developmental dilemma. Stern arrived at her interpretation of this phenomenon after studying contradictory theories of female adolescent development. On the one hand, some theorists take a purely developmental approach, emphasizing the psychological progress and change made during the adolescent phase of life, without particularly taking gender into account. Theorists in this camp emphasize the need boys and girls have

---

24. Stern, "Disavowing the Self," 108.
25. Stern, "Disavowing the Self," 108–9.

to establish identity and make independent decisions, tending to describe adolescence as a time of increasing separation — from parents, authority, convention. From this perspective, adolescence represents a steady gain in self-differentiation. Evidence of adolescent rebellion against authority supports this view of adolescence, yet it does not explain the disquieting silence and "ignorance" that can characterize female adolescence. On the other hand, some feminist theorists view adolescence from the perspective of women's shared experience. They tend to see it as the point when a girl acquires her nurturing and relational identity and her characteristic attentiveness and sensitivity to others. These theorists describe how during adolescence a girl typically adopts a sense of self that is contextual, relating herself to her place in the world of other persons. Adolescence, from this perspective, represents the enrichment of relationship.[26]

Stern decided that both types of theories were partially correct about the emotional and psychological tasks girls undertake during adolescence. She concluded that for girls, adolescence intensifies both the need to separate and the need to connect.[27] Thus, adolescence presents a girl with two different but equally important developmental tasks. This combination of tasks is especially difficult, however, because fulfilling one appears to conflict directly with fulfilling the other. This apparent conflict creates a dilemma for girls, and they attempt a response in disavowing the self, according to Stern. In other words, girls choose to disavow themselves as a way to straddle both horns of the dilemma: separation *and* connection, self-assertion *and* relationship. Instead of wrestling with the tension, they try to eliminate it and pretend that no dilemma exists.

A strategy of disavowal clearly has significant negative consequences for erotic life and, in particular, for decisions about sexual activity. This approach provides a way to interpret the lack of forthrightness in sexual situations that we heard girls voice in chapter 4. Despite the costs to

---

26. This type of psychological theory undergirds Carter Heyward's work. Heyward acknowledges her indebtedness to the Stone Center for Developmental Services and Studies at Wellesley College, and the Stone Center is known for its stress on the importance of empathy and empowerment in relationship. See Judith Jordan, "Empathy and the Mother-Daughter Relationship," in "Women and Empathy: Implications for Psychological Development and Psychotherapy," *Work in Progress,* no. 82–02 (Wellesley, Mass.: The Stone Center Working Paper Series, 1983); Janet L. Surrey, "Relationship and Empowerment," *Work in Progress,* no. 30 (Wellesley, Mass.: The Stone Center Working Paper Series, 1983); Jean Baker Miller, "What Do We Mean by Relationship?" *Work in Progress,* no. 22 (Wellesley, Mass.: The Stone Center Working Paper Series, 1986).

27. Adolescence tends to be different for boys, who do not necessarily experience the latter to the same degree, for reasons we note later in this chapter.

themselves of doing so, girls would apparently rather remain quiet about what they think and want than alienate their partners. Girls may also choose not to ratify their own inclinations and intentions in favor of acceding to their partners', in order not to alienate them. Indeed, Stern quotes Sheila, who made just such a choice:

> When my friend came down from California, he wanted to sleep together and I didn't want to, because at that point I felt like we were drifting apart and there wasn't that much left in it. It was a hard decision because if I had said that to him, obviously what's he going to say. "I'll be here forever, we'll always be together." That is obviously what he is going to say. And I probably would have fallen for it.[28]

Sheila knows her own resolve (not to sleep with him because they were drifting apart), but also knows that she would have let him convince her otherwise. She "solved" this contradiction by silencing her thoughts about what she wanted to do, which allowed her to keep her resolve while not acting according to it. In what Stern describes as a startlingly clear description of her dilemma, Sheila acknowledges the futility of her solution but also the reason it felt like the only one she had:

> It is like two people standing on a boat that they both know is sinking. I don't want to say anything to you because it will upset you, and you don't want to say anything to me because it will upset you. And we are both standing here in water up to our ankles watching it rise and I don't want to say anything to you.[29]

Stern's work further demonstrates why simple confidence in the erotic is an insufficient basis for a sexual ethic. Sustaining erotic relationships presents a challenge that liberating Eros will not in itself change. Many girls and women perceive a significant conflict, described vividly by Stern's Sheila, between preserving relationship and preserving self. Clearly this conflict is a deterrent to flourishing in erotic relationships. Girls and women cannot merely exercise more courage. They cannot simply adopt a more positive view of the erotic. One's sense of self and one's relationship to another are implicated in any expression of erotic passion. The

---

28. Stern, "Disavowing the Self," 110.
29. Stern, "Disavowing the Self," 111.

erotic lies precisely at the fulcrum of self-assertion and connection and easily turns into self-submission or self-aggrandizement when the balance is upset. Stern's work also puts us in search of a theory that will explain why asserting the self and connecting with others are crucially intertwined to begin with and why they are difficult to balance. Such a theory would explain why, for girls, being in relationship without disavowing the self is often a struggle. A theory like this would also lend greater clarity to the questions of how this struggle becomes gendered and why men's and women's ideas about the erotic are often constructed so differently. While also not a complete answer, feminist object relations theory can shed some helpful light on these issues.

Object Relations Theory

Object relations theory is a school of psychoanalytic thought that examines the formative bonds between an individual and significant persons in his or her life. All object relations theory centers on the claim that, above all else, the self is object-seeking. (Jane Flax calls this concept object relation's one essentialist claim.)[30] Among psychoanalytic theories, object relations theory is particularly useful because it interprets desires (erotic and otherwise) in terms of an individual self's relationship to significant objects and perceptions of objects. "Objects" refers to the symbolic psychic representations of persons; individuals' relationships to these objects are understood to be as important to their development as their relationships to the actual persons themselves. As the theory goes, soon after birth an individual's psyche begins to develop in relation to internalized memories, wishes, and fantasies of persons with whom it has formed significant bonds, especially mother and father. Alterations to these bonds, both positive and negative (e.g., death, estrangement, competition, adoption, sexual involvement, romantic love), chart the course of psychic development. Object relations theorists strive to explain the patterns in individuals' lives by analyzing their psyches both in relation to the social bonds they form with actual people and in relation to the internal psychic representations of those bonds. Jane Flax describes the school as follows: "Although object relations theorists differ somewhat among themselves, their overall

---

30. Jane Flax, *Thinking Fragments: Psychoanalysis, Feminism, and Postmodernism in the Contemporary West* (Berkeley: University of California Press, 1990), 111.

project is similar: to understand the 'individual' as the product of social relations with real persons in interaction with the unfolding development of his or her unique 'psyche-soma.'"[31]

Among object relations theorists, the work of Jessica Benjamin and Nancy Chodorow applies here because they have taken gender most seriously into account and have studied erotic bonding from social and cultural perspectives. Benjamin uses object relations theory to study patterns of domination and submission; Chodorow uses it to show how the inclination toward mothering continues to be "reproduced" in women and not men.[32]

Object relations theory traces back to Freud. In his early writings, Freud largely ignored the importance of objects in an individual's life. Looking primarily inward, he directed his interest toward the way individuals are driven to satisfy their desires and needs, with little regard to how these needs develop in relation to other people. He theorized further that the psyche develops as a child successfully satisfies his or her oral, anal, and genital needs — in that given order. These urges Freud called *instincts* or *drives;* he claimed that the individual instinctually seeks to obtain relief from the pent-up tension that these needs produced. This view of the desiring self did not particularly address who or what provides the relief. Drive theory reflected an assumption that the self is contained, private, and need-driven. In fact, drive theory almost suggested, as Flax points out, that if individuals could relieve their desires all by themselves, they wouldn't need other people.[33] In any event, this earlier view tended to reduce the role of other people in an individual's life to a functional, need-satisfying one.

Perhaps realizing the inadequacy of drive theory on its own, Freud came later to posit an additional way to understand the developing psyche, one that recognized the importance of bond formation in addition to need satisfaction. This became his object relations theory, which he de-

---

31. Flax, *Thinking Fragments,* 110. As a thinker and writer whose work spans philosophy, psychoanalytic practice, feminist thought, and political theory, Flax is especially well positioned to evaluate the discourses of these disciplines and examine their overlaps and gaps. Chapter 4 of *Thinking Fragments* provides a good summary of object relations theory and an endorsement of it over Lacanian theory in particular with respect to postmodern and feminist understandings of the self and social relations.

32. Jessica Benjamin, *Bonds of Love: Psychoanalysis, Feminism, and the Problem of Domination* (New York: Pantheon Books, 1988), and Nancy Chodorow, *The Reproduction of Mothering: Psychoanalysis and the Sociology of Gender* (Berkeley: University of California Press, 1978).

33. Flax, *Thinking Fragments,* 54.

veloped in "On Narcissism" (1914) and "The Ego and the Id" (1923). In these writings, Freud developed his theory of the ego and, in doing so, adopted a view of the self that is much more social and relational. The ego is essentially the collection of objects in which a person has ever significantly invested herself, emotionally and erotically, but has had to give up and thus internalize.[34] Therefore, Freud came to believe that the self is determined at least in part by the nature of its relationships to significant others, not only by drives or instincts. Actual relationships are internalized psychologically and carried within the person as important internal figures.

While one can study the object relations of any age, for us to study early childhood object relations is instructive because at least in part through them individuals learn fundamental lessons about their own needs, interests, and passions and about how these factors are integrated into their relationships with other persons. The groundwork for identity and self-esteem is laid at an early age, as are the emotional and psychological skills of succeeding in relationship. Interpersonal patterns and practices that people adopt as adults can often be traced to the nature of their early object relations. Indeed, many of the emotional and psychological struggles that people go through during adolescence and adulthood represent renewals of struggles left over from early childhood. Nancy Chodorow argues that the study of early childhood object relations is important to an understanding of the interpersonal dynamics of later life for at least three reasons: Persons develop their basic psychological orientation to their interpersonal world during infancy and childhood; persons emerge from childhood with strong memories of deep interpersonal bonds (which they often attempt to re-create); and impressions of gender, and their import for interpersonal relations, are deeply imprinted during the first years of life.[35]

Object relations theory is not without its critics, especially among stricter neo-Freudian theorists and Lacanians, and particularly regarding the subject of the erotic. I will not enter those specific debates.[36] Within the feminist community, however, three criticisms relevant to this project

---

34. Sigmund Freud, "The Ego and the Id," in *Complete Psychological Works of Sigmund Freud*, trans. and ed. James Strachey, vol. 19 (London: The Hogarth Press, 1957), 29.

35. Chodorow, *The Reproduction of Mothering*, 57.

36. I will say, however, that I do not use Lacan because he explains desire in entirely linguistic terms and is not a developmentalist at all. His notion of erotic "desire" is not necessarily object-related. I do not use stricter neo-Freudian theorists because they continue to view the self as

arise frequently: that object relations theories are universalistic, that they are essentialist, and that they are deterministic. People who level the first critique say that object relations theories, like psychoanalytic theories in general, make unwarranted claims to universalism, especially with respect to gender and family. Benjamin and Chodorow, though, developed their object relations theories from observations of a specific type of family (however common), namely, the traditional gender-structured family in which the mother assumes primary care of young children and the father assumes the role of breadwinner. Their theories apply only to persons who grew up in this type of family with its cultural patterns.[37] Jessica Benjamin writes: "Only in Western middle-class families do we see the typical pattern of babies attended by one lone mother. Thus our theory, unless amended, might strictly apply to such families."[38] In other words, the psychological patterns she and Chodorow describe are to some extent socially and culturally specific, and they both acknowledge that different contexts would produce different patterns; so their theories, at least, are not falsely universalistic. At the same time, the division of labor just described is still a very common one within the American family; hence the claims of object relations theorists that their observations apply to a great many Americans are still warranted. Furthermore, their theories need not be restricted to people who were actually raised by a mother-father pair, for the father or mother "object" can still be present even if the actual person is absent.[39]

People who level the second critique charge that in assuming an inherent human interest in forming relational bonds (and particularly with one's mother), object relations theorists make essentialist claims that define human life too narrowly and precisely. Inarguably, these theories ought to be open to the diverse ways that people's interpersonal lives are constructed. But nothing in the theories themselves prevents this approach.

---

primarily need-driven and therefore do not sufficiently appreciate the impact of the self's actual, social relations with others in the world.

37. This type of family is not only specified with respect to gender but also with respect to class and race. That is, generally only in contemporary Western middle- and upper-class families can parents even afford to divide the child-rearing and breadwinning roles; generally only in white families are the roles of child rearing and breadwinning so closely identified with the mother and father alone.

38. Benjamin, *Bonds of Love,* 75.

39. Chodorow's work seems to me even less open to the charge of false universalism because she limits herself to studying (only) girls who grow up to mother after having themselves been mothered by women.

As long as one accepts that bond formation is psychologically significant in human life (a rather minimal claim) and that what happens in early childhood affects what happens in adulthood (likewise relatively minimal), object relations theory can apply to a wide variety of human situations and conditions.[40] Moreover, feminist object relations theorists are committed to examining the interplay of social structures, gender roles, and psychology and therefore steadfastly avoid many essentialist claims in order to highlight the constructed nature of gender development.

Finally, some people contend that object relations theorists try to determine how individuals will "turn out" while ignoring other factors in human life such as biology and culture. However, like all psychoanalytic theories, object relations theory presents itself as but one way to understand how individuals become who they are and does not preclude other ways. Social and cultural influences, as well as biological imperatives, combine with the inclinations of the psyche to construct human behavior in complex ways. Unlike drive theories or linguistic theories, in fact, object relations theories acknowledge this complexity and take into account how the configuration of actual human relationships (especially the family) builds individual selves.[41]

One way to summarize these replies to the critics is to say that object relations theory remains consistent with a constructionist view of self and experience while restraining any extreme move in a postmodernist direction. According to object relations theory, the self is a product of social bonds and human community; that is, object relations theory posits a contextual and localized self rather than a transcendent, ahistorical one and is therefore compatible with social constructionist theories. Critical theorist Seyla Benhabib, for example, borrows object relations language in defending her "post-metaphysical universalist" view of the human person as finite and fragile over against the disembodied cogito of the Enlightenment:

40. One example of such an application is Chodorow's book *Femininities, Masculinities, Sexualities: Freud and Beyond,* in which she questions the normative status of heterosexuality and examines gender variations within romantic love (Lexington, Ky.: The University Press of Kentucky, 1994).
41. Benjamin, Chodorow, and others are clinicians as well as academicians; their theories are grounded not only in intellectual work but also in their work with clients. This fact helps to temper any tendency toward false universalism. As Chodorow writes, "[m]y increasing certainty about the importance of context, specificity, and personal individuality grows principally not from [my readings of psychoanalytic texts] but from my clinical observations of the extraordinary uniqueness, complexity, and particularity of any individual psyche," *Femininities, Masculinities, Sexualities,* ix–x.

The human infant becomes a "self," a being capable of speech and action, only by learning to interact in a human community. The self becomes an individual in that it becomes a "social" being capable of language, interaction and cognition. The identity of the self is constituted by a narrative unity, which integrates what "I" can do, have done and will accomplish with what you expect of "me," interpret my acts and intentions to mean, wish for me in the future, etc.[42]

At the same time, the self of object relations, while contingent upon the specificities of its historical narrative, retains coherence. The self is not dispersed into myriad social relations and interactions. "I" have a distinct identity and can interpret and effect change in my world. In fact, grounded as object relations theory is in the therapeutic realm, one of its primary aims is to assist people in interpreting and remedying their own dysfunctional patterns and practices so that they might live better lives. Therefore, this particular theory avoids the dangers of nihilism and relativism that can beset postmodern theories.

Attachment and Separation

For persons to invest themselves in meaningful, intimate relationships with others without forfeiting their own sense of self is not at all easy. The dual challenge of connection and separation characterizes even the mother-infant bond, often lifted up as the paradigmatically blissful human relationship. Mother and infant are not spared the difficulty of figuring out how to get what they each want and stay true to themselves without completely disregarding the other and losing their shared intimacy. Indeed, relationships of blissful union hardly come naturally to the human psyche. While they add immense richness to life, they do not come without some cost to the strong, independent self. Any intimate human relationship is the product of a delicate balancing of connection and separation, as we shall see, and represents a rare treasure in human life.

The development of a person's sense of self — and correspondingly, a sense of how to relate to others — begins when an infant learns that it is separate from its mother.[43] An infant has to learn this, the argument goes,

---

42. Seyla Benhabib, *Situating the Self: Gender, Community, and Postmodernism in Contemporary Ethics* (New York: Routledge, 1992), 5.

43. Two notes about language: Following the theorists I employ, I will call the primary caregiver the mother. While it might be more precise to use "primary caregiver" each time, in the culture I am studying — contemporary American society — most often the primary caregiver *is*

because at first the infant does not distinguish itself from its mother. But at some point after birth, the infant discovers that what seems like one self is really two. Until then, the infant does not really understand that nourishment and touch and care come from outside itself, and hence it experiences its body and self as continuous with its mother's. Since its needs are consistently met, the infant does not actually experience them as needs.[44] Nevertheless, the mother's care builds in the infant a sense of security and self-coherence and thus the rudimentary foundations of selfhood. An infant who can trust in care and consistency does not have to concern itself with survival, does not have to adapt to unfavorable conditions, and can flourish and begin to "experience [it]self as an effective emotional and interpersonal agent."[45] In contrast, an infant that experiences intermittent care does not know to "blame" an outsider and consequently doubts the effectiveness of its own agency. If its mother were to respond totally randomly to its expressions of need, the infant would feel a sense of fragmentation and incoherence and would eventually develop uncertainty about itself. In other words, from the very beginning of life, an infant's developing sense of self is dialectically related to the responses of its primary caregiver.

As an infant matures and is able to initiate actions, its developing self continues to depend on seeing itself mirrored in others. In simple and concrete terms, a child learns, for example, that its smiles evoke smiles from the others it knows, that another entity can mimic the child's cooing or arm-waving or restlessness. Developmentalists explain that a child actually needs to have its actions and feelings consistently mirrored, or at

the mother. The fact that women do the primary caregiving is also an important factor in the development of gender difference, and hence emphasizing the gender of the primary caregiver is appropriate. To adopt gender neutrality in my language, in other words, would actually be misleading. Also following these theorists, I call the infant "it" even though this may sound strange to the ear. The reason for this is likewise to avoid falsely gendered language — in this case, to avoid attributing gender before gender becomes a significant developmental issue. I start using gendered pronouns when I start talking about gender differentiation.

44. These claims are no longer universally accepted. They were pioneered by Margaret Mahler during the 1960s. Mahler created the concept of the "psychological birth of the human infant," referring to the recognition of selfhood. She believed that the realization that one self has become two — a kind of psychological "birth" — did not occur until at least four or five months into life. Not until then, she argued, does an infant realize that it is separate from its mother. See Margaret Mahler, Fred Pine, and Anni Bergmann, *The Psychological Birth of the Human Infant* (New York: Basic Books, 1975). Many theorists still accept this claim while others do not. Nevertheless, a successful process of self-development appears to depend on experiences both of bonding and of separation and not necessarily on the timing of first separation.

45. Chodorow, *The Reproduction of Mothering*, 60.

least responded to, to learn that it can author them at all. If no one else ever shared one's intentions and emotions, they might be experienced as random and chaotic and therefore, ironically, not really one's own. Jessica Benjamin puts it this way:

> A person comes to feel that "I am the doer who does, I am the author of my acts," by being with another person who recognizes her acts, her feelings, her intentions, her existence, her independence. Recognition is the essential response, the constant companion of assertion. The subject declares, "I am, I do," and then waits for the response, "You are, you have done."[46]

As Benjamin explains, to develop as a self, an individual cannot just make the assertive declaration, "I am, I do." Full authority for one's being and doing does not depend on greater independence from others but actually requires an audience who can declare, "You are, you have done."

In order to feel authoritative and coherent, and to be able to name and claim our own experiences, in other words, we have to be able to trust that the actions we initiate and the passions we express will evoke responses from our community of others. At the same time, however, we also must be able to trust that the actions we initiate are ours, not theirs. The psychic problem of the relationship between self and other becomes complex at this point. Acquiring a sense of self may depend on connecting with others, but clearly the two tasks also compete at some level. One can risk losing either awareness of others or awareness of self. To become differentiated, to become a distinct and separate individual, may require that one stay in relation to others — but differentiation will never happen if one simply merges one's self with theirs. And the converse is also true: A stable relationship depends on the existence of two distinct and separate selves even while each self owes itself, in a sense, to the other.

Thus, we can already see that even at the earliest stage in life, staying in relationship creates contradiction and, at times, conflict for an individual. The dual fantasy of utter devotion and triumphant detachment compete at a fundamental level. While the infant may fantasize that the mother should serve its every need and desire, it also wants to remain separate from her. Balancing the needs for both attachment and separation is the goal, but like any dialectic, achieving balance is not easy.

---

46. Benjamin, *Bonds of Love*, 21.

We should note that when the right balance is successfully struck —
when both partners to a relationship are both assertive and yielding —
genuine "mutuality" is achieved. "Mutual" relationships are not perfectly
blissful unions; quite the contrary, they always display an amount of psychic tension. Mutuality should not be idealized as a condition of utter
devotion and harmony, but rather valued as a quality of relationship with
a continual striving for balance. This factor is important to remember
when mutuality is lifted up as a virtue in feminist theologies of the erotic.

As a baby grows older, the potential contradiction between attachment
and separation intensifies as different developmental tasks present themselves. Self-consciousness — that is, the awareness that others have access
to one's own subjective states — develops during the first year of life. An
infant begins to realize that people can share thinking and emotion, which
were previously experienced as entirely subjective. This discovery can be
pleasurable for the infant.

> This conscious pleasure in sharing a feeling introduces a new level
> of mutuality — a sense that inner experience can be joined, that two
> minds can cooperate in one intention. This conception of emerging
> intersubjectivity emphasizes how the awareness of the separate other
> enhances the felt connection with him: this *other* mind can share *my*
> feeling.[47]

Theorists agree that the pleasure of this reciprocal attunement prefigures
adult eroticism; in other words, part of the gratification of erotic experience stems from its potential to fulfill deep fantasies of being completely
attuned to another.

The pleasure of intersubjectivity is offset, however, by the need to
become more independent. This need ironically also corresponds to the
discovery of self-consciousness: The child begins to experience a strong
urge to wrest itself free of sharing everything, and identifying so closely,
with another. (Correspondingly, another feature of adult eroticism can be
the exciting "tension" produced by alterity and even opposition.) At about
fourteen months, children enter the phase that psychoanalysts call rapprochement, a phase marked by friction and paradox. In rapprochement
the child starts seriously to seek independence, while at the same time still
basking in the assurance of its mother's devotion. The child continues to

---

47. Benjamin, *Bonds of Love*, 30.

have fantasies of being one with her, but it also begins to fantasize about the utter opposite, having complete control *over* her. As a way to pry itself free from bonds that are starting to feel confining, the rapprochement child fantasizes that it is omnipotent and that all others exist for it. Yet at the same time, the child does not want the boundaries between itself and others to be erased, for others must remain a readily available audience. Both are important. This paradox means significant internal indecision about the relative value of separateness versus attachment. Hence, rapprochement can be a traumatic time psychologically for the child — and for family members as well, who experience the child as increasingly demanding and even impertinent. (Freud dubbed the rapprochement child "His Majesty the Baby," reflecting the willfullness of this stage.)

Rapprochement psychodynamics graphically demonstrate the difficult dilemma in human life of simultaneously wanting to discover who one is and to assert oneself and wanting to accommodate others whom one loves. Issues of possession, control, and surrender predominate and significantly test mother-child relationships during this period. The danger lies in either party "winning" the battle for independence. From the child's perspective, two psychodynamics are possible: The child may attempt to assume the mother-object into itself to seize independence, or the child may attempt to subsume itself into her to remain connected. Benjamin describes these alternative fantasies:

> The child may be tempted to believe that the other person is not separate. ("She belongs to me, I control and possess her.") In short, he fails to confront his own dependency on someone outside himself. Alternatively, the child may continue to see the mother as all-powerful, and [her]self as helpless. In this case, the apparent acceptance of dependency masks the effort to retain control by remaining connected to the mother ("I am good and powerful because I am exactly like my good and powerful mother wishes me to be"). This child does not believe [s]he will ever gain recognition for [her] own independent self, and so [s]he denies that self.[48]

Thus, we can already see how the seeds are sown of disavowal of self during female adolescence. Not unlike rapprochement children, fe-

---

48. Benjamin, *Bonds of Love,* 52–53. I have changed Benjamin's pronouns in the latter part of the paragraph to reflect the gender difference she argues for.

male adolescents (and many of the rest of us) are highly ambivalent about independence and dependence, wanting at the same time to become "their own people" and also to maintain or establish intimacy with others. Two ways to resolve the contradiction are available, and one lies in (apparent) acceptance of dependency. One gives up on being recognized, disavows the self, and opts for identifying with the more powerful other. The question remains as to why the female psyche tends to resolve the contradiction this way. After all, as Benjamin notes, another option is to refuse to admit separateness by controlling and possessing the other. But as we shall see, the genders tend to diverge in the strategies they adopt. Under conditions of female parenting in a gender-structured family, girls tend to opt for disavowal — or less drastically, for defining their identities and passions out of their close identification with "good and powerful others." Boys tend to reject such close identification because of the dependency it represents and prefer "having" others instead. The implications for erotic experience can be significant. If one chooses disavowal and complete identification with the other, one will likely express eroticism in terms of surrender and merger. One's ideas about what is exciting and pleasurable may be built around attunement, identification, and even submission. Conversely, if one prefers domination and utter difference from the other, one's erotic "repertoire" will form around domination and possession.

Gender-Differentiated Relationships

We come now to considering directly the role of gender. The question of when gender difference begins to have an impact on development is a difficult question to answer with precision, since boys' and girls' experiences likely diverge from the very start. That is, many theorists argue that male and female children receive differential treatment from the moment of birth and hence begin from day one to develop differently according to gender.[49] Nevertheless, gender eventually comes to have a known

---

49. While consensus around this theory may be growing, differential treatment during early infancy and childhood nevertheless remains difficult to prove. That is, proving that mothers and fathers handle and treat their young sons and daughters differently is difficult. Some researchers claim that differential treatment is even impossible to demonstrate empirically. Chodorow argues that while such differentiation may not be provable, it is plausible. She extrapolates backwards from clinical observations of patients whose histories suggest friction in the maternal-infant relationship, and she hypothesizes that, in general, different patterns tend to emerge from mother-daughter relationships than mother-son ones.

and direct impact on object relations when children become aware that their mothers are female persons. When they begin to be aware of their mothers' gender, and correspondingly learn their own gender, girls' and boys' relationships with their mothers — and the strategies with which they defend their own emerging sense of self — begin to diverge.

Somewhere between eighteen and twenty-four months, a child learns its gender, which is to say that she learns that she is a girl, like her mother, and not a boy, like her father.[50] Learning gender is part of the general process of establishing particular and unique personhood, which is called "differentiation" because the young child is focused on differentiating its personality from others'. Through differentiation, a child develops a unique and full-blown identity of its own. At this stage, its sense of self is constructed out of the growing knowledge of its idiosyncratic preferences, skills, experiences, desires, and memories. The child increasingly experiences these features as unique to itself, as indeed they usually are. In addition, the child learns that it is different from some others (and similar to other others) by virtue of its gender.

The most significant person from whom the child has to differentiate itself is its primary caretaker, usually its mother. She is the person the child is naturally inclined to think it is most like. The child's and mother's sense of oneness, described earlier, creates this inclination. The child thus knows no better than to think that it will become like her in all ways.[51] Chodorow explains why in many families, even before gender becomes important, neither girls nor boys necessarily think they will become like their fathers:

> Fathers often become external attachment figures for children of both genders during their preoedipal years. But the intensity and exclusivity of the relationship is much less than with a mother, and fathers are from the outset separate people and "special." As a result, representations of the father relationship do not become . . . so

---

50. I use "gender" as nearly synonymous for "sex" here, although I realize that some feminists would insist on different language to stress the social construction of gender. Nevertheless, to learn one's biological sex *is* to learn one's social gender in a society that constructs social and cultural types out of sex differences. A little girl does not merely learn that she has a vulva, but learns that having a vulva puts her with her mother in a distinctive social group that is different from the group her brother and father are in.

51. Were the child genuinely to have several equally significant caretakers, its object relations would be different and probably the task of differentiation would be as well.

determining of the person's identity and sense of self, as do representations of the relationship to a mother.[52]

But, of course, not all children become like their mother in all ways. Some become boys. To grasp the difference between boys' and girls' differentiation, then, is to see that in traditional gender-structured families, boys and girls both differentiate themselves from a female person. Hence, the psychodynamics of gender acquisition are different for each: Becoming a girl is different from becoming a boy. Boys learn that they are unlike their mother while girls learn that they are like her. To become a girl is to become a similar kind of person to one's primary love object while to become a boy is to become a different kind of person from one's primary love object.

We can put it another way: Predominantly female parenting means that learning gender identity becomes a process either of discovering similarity or of discovering dissimilarity, either identification or disidentification. "Identification" is not merely an acknowledgment of shared interests and history but a technical term for an intense love relationship. For infants, to "identify with" the mother means to forge the bonds of recognition, dependence, and trust that I spoke of earlier. The meaning of identification retains this sense of intimacy and intensity even for an older child. Thus, male gender differentiation, as a process of disidentification, involves at least in part a repudiation of this intense love relationship and of the boy's bond with his mother.

The two psychodynamic processes — identification and disidentification — may be complementary, but they are unequal. For a boy to accomplish adequate separation from his mother, as mother and as female, he must make certain claims to discontinuity and difference. Object relations theorists argue that continuing to identify with someone is not as great a task as disidentifying with them. For a boy to learn eventually that he is, in an important way, unlike his mother is a significant — even traumatic — experience. (For this reason, many psychoanalysts actually view gender differentiation as more of a psychological hurdle for boys than girls.) Therefore, a boy may ironically try to resolve the difficulty of staying connected to his mother while growing apart from her by denying

---

52. Chodorow, *The Reproduction of Mothering*, 96–97. If the father were the primary caregiver, then presumably the mother would be the external attachment figure, and the father-child relationship more constitutive of the child's identity.

his connection to her. As Benjamin puts it: "The premise of his independence is to say, 'I am nothing like she who cares for me.'"[53] The tension in becoming a self, requiring both differentiation and attachment, reduces to the former pole for boys, and differentiation becomes the paramount way of establishing who they are. In certain contexts, a son may fantasize about ceasing to relate to his mother at all, and differentiation becomes disavowal of the other.

Girls, on the other hand, do not generally need to make these same claims to discontinuity. Gender identity comes more easily for a girl, according to this theory, because identifying with the mother is continuous. Acquiring a female identity does not necessitate a girl's staking psychological distance from her mother. Thus, little girls are spared some of the anguish that boys go through at this time. But while girls may not have the same challenge of loosening the bond with their mothers to establish their gender, they nonetheless still have the problem of adequately differentiating themselves. Ironically, because the girl does not need to fantasize about rejecting her mother, she may not do enough psychological work to differentiate herself, that is, to avow herself as a distinct and separate person. Benjamin writes:

> Whereas the boy's early difficulty seems to occur in making the switch to a masculine identification, the girl requires no such shift in identification away from her mother. This makes her identity less problematic, but it is a disadvantage in that she possesses no obvious way of disidentifying from her mother, no hallmark of separateness. The feminine tendency therefore is not to emphasize but to underplay independence.[54]

A girl may therefore find it difficult to recognize herself as truly separate, to ease psychologically and emotionally away from her mother, and to assert her sense of self. In contrast to a boy's fantasy, a girl might fantasize, "I am everything like she who cares for me." The tension between differentiation and attachment may reduce to the pole of attachment. The girl knows who she is by knowing to whom she is attached. In some cases, she may develop a tendency to disavow herself.

We can thus appreciate how the seeds are sown for female adolescent

---

53. Benjamin, *Bonds of Love*, 76.
54. Benjamin, *Bonds of Love*, 78.

disavowal of self and preoccupation with relationship. According to the object relations theory we have been tracing, girls' psychic strategies for resolving the paradox of needing both separation and attachment incline them toward the latter. Early on, girls figure out ways to construct a sense of self that has built into it, as it were, being part of another so that they can remain separate selves while still attached. All the issues associated with attachment and relationship — closeness, attunement, oneness — thus become central preoccupations for girls. They form the meaning of being a self in relationship. Object relations theorists argue that girls continue to be preoccupied with issues of relationship for an even longer time during early childhood than boys do. A girl may continue longer than a boy, for example, to try to re-create the blissful oneness she had with her mother as an infant.

Remember that these generalizations hold only within particular familial contexts. Predominantly female parenting is one important factor. If girls and boys were cared for equally by mother and father (or, for that matter, by two mothers, two fathers, or yet some other familial arrangement) and treated the same by parents and others, their developmental journeys might look quite different. These generalizations likewise gloss over particularities such as the sturdiness of the mother's own object relations, the mother's and father's marriage (or lack thereof), family traumas, and the nature of sibling relationships. All of these factors combine to create an individual's own unique history of object relations; no two psyches are exactly alike. Nevertheless, the point is that when parenting roles are structured along gender lines, with mother and father representing contrasting symbols of love and desire, and contrasting ways of negotiating the tensions of intimacy, that structure colors the picture of children's development in not insignificant ways. This arrangement ties gender into the problems of interpersonal relationship at a very deep level. Far-reaching effects include the way erotic experience is constructed later in life. We see these effects continuing to build in the next stage of development, the oedipal period.

Oedipal Relationships

To see how gender differences in self-development and relationship are further aggravated, we must examine the final significant hurdle of early childhood development, the so-called Oedipus complex. The Oedipus complex is a psychological process that both male and female children go through sometime around the third year of life. In classical theory, the (male) child is forced to acknowledge that while he adores his mother, he cannot have her all to himself because he must share her with his father. To resolve the psychic tension of hating his father for this and wanting to possess his mother, he trades these feelings in for the status of being his father's pride and joy and his mother's second love. His complex thus resolved, he assumes his rightful place in the family as his father's son and mother's little man. Feminist object relations theorists modify this narrative to include daughters and to unseat its sexist assumptions.[55] Consistent with their psychoanalytic interests, feminist object relations theorists look not just at how the girls' and boys' psyches fare during the oedipal stage, but also at how their object relations fare — what this phase confirms for them about being in relationship. Consistent with their feminism, they look particularly at how the struggles of the oedipal period lay the groundwork for female disavowal of self, female orientation toward relationality, and female perplexity about erotic desiring.

The first thing object relations theorists emphasize is that oedipal relationships are not discontinuous with earlier phases in development but represent their continuation. As we have already seen, whether male or female, a child's relationship to its mother is fraught with intensity and ambivalence because of the difficulty of maintaining attachment without risking lack of differentiation, and vice versa. Any relationship characterized by both intensity and ambivalence cannot be sustained for long without relief. The shift to oedipal relationships provides this relief. A little boy recovers from his earlier trauma of separating from his mother during the oedipal phase by solidifying his relationship with his father. He discovers in his father a figure in whom he can recognize himself and receive affirmation of his maleness. (This state is called identification, or identificatory love.) His relationship with his mother correspondingly shifts; from being someone he wants to become, she becomes someone he aims to have. Part of identifying with his father is identifying with his

---

55. Feminist psychoanalytic theorists like Benjamin and Chodorow, as well as others like Melanie Klein and Janine Chasseguet-Smirgel before them, have done substantial work to revise Freud's presentation of the Oedipus complex, especially by focusing on the nature of oedipal relationships rather than the consequences of oedipal drives. See Melanie Klein, "Early Stages of the Oedipus Conflict," *International Journal of Psycho-Analysis* 9 (1928): 67–180, and *The Psychoanalysis of Children* (London: Hogarth Press, 1959); and Janine Chasseguet-Smirgel, "Outline for a Study of Narcissism in Female Sexuality," in *Female Sexuality,* ed. Chasseguet-Smirgel (Ann Arbor: University of Michigan Press, 1970). Benjamin and Chodorow go beyond early theorists in challenging the gendered assumptions of classical (Freudian) theory.

father's love relationship to his mother; and so while not sharing precisely the same love, the son's adoration of his mother becomes protective and possessive rather than needy and vulnerable. He learns, if you will, to love her as a male loves a female. His separation from his primary love object thus reinforced and reconfigured, he joins the male world of agency and power.

Little girls, too, try to identify with the exciting, powerful father figure to resolve their own needs for relief from the intense mother-daughter bond. During the oedipal phase, they too yearn for an identificatory love relationship with the father. They see in their fathers potential for escape from the maternal world. Feminist psychoanalytic theorists call this the "turn to the father."[56] Unfortunately, however, girls are not received into relationship by their fathers the same way their brothers are. For many girls, moreover, fathers are not ready identificatory figures. Fathers typically tend not to let their daughters identify with them by treating their daughters as different, precious, and vulnerable objects. Consequently, fathers ironically reinforce their own status as distant, unavailable love objects. As a result, a girl's attempt at identification with and separation via her father during the oedipal phase, while significant, is generally less successful than a boy's. She ends up falling back upon the bond she has established with her mother.

In the end, the oedipal phase leaves girls with the same kind of psychic grief that the differentiation phase left for boys, and girls remain snarled in issues of separation and differentiation to which the maternal-child bond has given rise. They are also less successful in learning how to love another through identifying with them and as a result fall back on the idealizing love they know so well from the maternal relationship. Benjamin (whose primary interest, we recall, is in how patterns of domination develop) explains:

---

56. Traditionally, this condition has been called "penis envy." Benjamin concedes that the oedipal phenomenon Freud termed "penis envy" does occur in young girls but has a better explanation than Freud supplied. Freud thought that at three years of age, girls suddenly discover that they lack penises, reject their mothers in dismay at this discovery, and turn to their fathers to try to obtain the desired genitalia. Benjamin acknowledges the yearning for the father captured in this scenario, but suggests a better explanation than by positing sudden genital envy. She argues instead that it represents a girl's attempt finally to achieve separation from her sometimes stifling identification with her mother by identifying ever more vigorously with her father. The phenomenon given the name "penis envy" may therefore be genuine, but is best understood as the logical result of the struggle to separate from the mother.

When identificatory love succeeds in toddlerhood, accompanied by the pleasure of mutual recognition, then identification can serve as a vehicle for developing one's own agency and desire. But when identificatory love is not satisfied within this context of mutual recognition — as it frequently is not for girls — it later emerges as ideal love, the wish for a vicarious substitute for one's own agency.[57]

Clearly implications exist here for erotic desire. Many girls emerge from toddlerhood with an association between romantic love and passive adoration or even unrequited longing. Because they have resorted to relationships of idealizing love, they may find later in life that pining away or even submitting to another's desire is "erotic."

Chodorow argues that the incomplete resolution of the oedipal phase accounts for the way girls develop "relational potential." Girls' sense of self has built into it, as it were, a sense of connecting and attuning to others. "The basic feminine sense of self is connected to the world, the basic masculine sense of self is separate."[58] Being half of a dyad, even where girls are the more dependent half, comes increasingly easily to them. In technical terms, the objects to which a girl is related become more fixed inside her ego because relating to an object (her mother) was a more profound and continuous part of her early experience. (Note that I am now speaking of a special feature of the postoedipal female self, not the fundamental inclination to relate and bond to others that object relations theory says all persons share *qua* persons.) In contrast, a boy's sense of self tends to be achieved through claims of difference, distance, and separation.

Object relations theory does not necessarily lead us to the conclusion that relationality is better (or worse, for that matter) than individuality, only that relationality is half of what a healthy ego needs. Object relations theory does not applaud girls' psychic strategies any more than it does boys'. Many feminists, including some feminist theologians of the erotic, say that we should celebrate women's special potential for relationality and the corresponding virtues of empathy, awareness of others, and so forth to which it gives rise. While I agree that these capacities are valuable in human life, I do not think they should be uncritically val-

---

57. Benjamin, *Bonds of Love*, 122.
58. Chodorow, *The Reproduction of Mothering*, 169.

orized.[59] To be so continually attuned to another's needs and interests that one ignores one's own is not a recipe for flourishing, according to either object relations theory or a feminist agenda. To be so interested in oneness and merger that one fails to differentiate oneself does not foster self-confidence and the ability to assert oneself. To favor dependence over interdependence as a way to achieve "mutuality" does not promote salutary relationships. In short, far from idealizing them, psychoanalytic theory reminds us that these female tendencies are potentially dangerous to healthy self-development and healthy relationship. In erotic life, they can lead as easily to harmful patterns and practices as they can to fulfillment.

A second important aspect of oedipal relationships helps to explain not only why girls disavow themselves and become preoccupied with relationship, but also why they are seemingly unable to claim their own thoughts and feelings. In traditional gender-structured families, and in the culture at large, the father not only represents an alternative love object (to the mother) for his young children, but also the one with more independence and power relative to the mother. Thus, he is an important provider of the necessary mirroring and response for children's intentions and desires that we considered earlier. The father is in a unique position to validate the developing child's sense of agency and passion simply because he himself represents agency and passion.[60] Indeed, in explaining a girl's oedipal "turn to the father," Benjamin goes beyond Chodorow to argue that a girl does not merely turn to him because he is the next available figure to help her escape from the maternal relationship. She argues that a girl's father represents something that she perceives her mother to lack and that she herself admires: agency.

The reason she admires it is because issues of agency have become increasingly crucial by age two. The child has moved beyond simply wanting to have her needs met and her desires satisfied. She now wants validation for her very wanting as well. She wants to be recognized as an agent

---

59. Nor do I think that they should be identified as an essence of womanhood. To conclude from psychoanalytic arguments about early childhood that women are "naturally" or "biologically" inclined to seek relationship or to care about others is incorrect. Freud often used naturalistic language, especially when writing about women, but his followers have since shown that psychoanalytic theory does not depend on such claims. Instead, the theoretical conclusions that I have been drawing depend on particular social configurations of family (the opposite of "natural") and, hence, the particular object relations that develop in those families.

60. Such claims need not be taken literally to have validity. In other words, I am not claiming that all fathers are more passionate than all mothers. A father figure can stand for passion without enacting it.

who wills and desires things. Benjamin describes the twenty-month-old in these terms:

> Nothing is more characteristic of this phase than the reiteration of the word "want." Where the fourteen-month-old said "banana" or "cracker" and pointed, the twenty-month-old says "Want that!" uninterested in naming the object itself. Recognition of this wanting is now the essential meaning of getting what you asked for.[61]

The child turns to the person she perceives as having the greatest power to name and satisfy *his* desires because she believes this person will best be able to recognize *her* own emerging ones. Again, however, little girls come to grief over this needed recognition; fathers are generally less available to them and, when they are, more likely to see them as adorable and vulnerable than to acknowledge the strength of their passion and desires.[62] This oedipal issue therefore goes unresolved as well, and girls' declarations of "Want that!" go unrecognized. Undoubtedly, boys may frequently experience occasions in which they do not receive the things they want and consequently feel frustrated. But in contrast to his sister, a boy's basic experience of wanting something is validated. His desires garner attention, whether or not they are ultimately satisfied. In addition, a boy believes that his father, the person he is coming to identify with, gets what *he* wants much of the time.

A boy thus comes to feel that he is *entitled* to desire things while a girl may not. She may even be actively discouraged from naming her desires. And so where the boy feels frustrated, the girl feels perplexed. A boy may be told, "No, you don't get x," but a girl is told, "You shouldn't ask for x," which is a more confusing message and more devastating to her self-confidence. Eventually, a girl whose desiring is ignored might come to question, at some level, her own desiring. In short, the less successful oedipal turn to the father may contribute to the risk girls face later in life of being tentative, compliant, and even confused about what they know and want.

---

61. Benjamin, *Bonds of Love*, 101.
62. Sometimes mothers exacerbate this frustration by projecting onto their daughters their own unrecognized wants and desires, considering daughters extensions of themselves and thus failing to provide the needed recognition.

Ideas Carried into Adolescence

Our discussion of object relations has shown that even before they reach the age of engaging in erotic activity, girls' ideas about the erotic have been formed from the matrix of intimate relationships they have already experienced. If adolescent girls have grown up in traditional gender-structured families, they have likely experienced a protracted period of intense and exclusive bonding with one parent, less opportunity than boys for psychological separation and individual differentiation, and insufficient affirmation for being a passionate person and female at the same time. They enter adolescence with a nexus of ideas (whether they are aware of them or not) about relationship and a set of dispositions and preoccupations that have been forming since early childhood. We can extrapolate from what Chodorow says about the reproduction of mothering to the reproduction of female eroticism:

> Women develop capacities for mothering from their object-relational stance. This stance grows out of the special nature and length of their preoedipal relationship to their mother; the nonabsolute repression of oedipal relationships; and their general ongoing mother-daughter preoccupation as they are growing up. It also develops because they have not formed the same defenses against relationship as men.[63]

As many women develop capacities for mothering, many girls develop capacities for compliance, idealization of the other, disavowal of self, attentiveness, and connection. These become girls' capacities for erotic relating; or, to put it another way, they constitute "erotic" behavior for girls in our culture (the way that caring and nurturing constitute mothering). For many girls, then, that "eroticism" is defined by intense romantic intimacy, pleasing a partner, dreamy visions of blissful union, perhaps even submission should come as no great surprise. These images are not only picked up from popular culture (though they certainly find reinforcement there), but they also represent the way girls are psychologically primed within their family life to think about erotic relationship.

Carrying these inchoate but powerful ideas about the meaning of the erotic with them into adolescence, girls attempt to negotiate sexual involvement on their terms, often to meet with more difficulty. They quickly discover that sexuality and the erotic mean quite different things to others.

---

63. Chodorow, *The Reproduction of Mothering*, 204.

They hear conflicting moral messages about who may have sex and for what reasons. They encounter new ideas, some appealing and some repellent, and struggle to incorporate these concepts into their sense of who they are and who they want to become. In particular, many ideas are thrust at them about what being sexual and a girl means. Meanwhile, they cannot shake completely from their minds the assumptions about sexuality and femininity that are lodged there, even if they no longer really subscribe to them and want to embrace different ideals and act in different ways.

Above all, girls leave the relatively serene world of childhood and enter the new world of adolescence — a world of double standards, sexist judgments, unsolicited attention, and heightened pressure to conform to gender roles and logics. Aware of these conflicts, but relatively powerless to resolve them, teenage girls are rarely able to negotiate erotic relationships that bring the kind of fulfillment they (think they) want. As we have seen in this chapter, individuals have difficulty changing even their own thoughts and feelings about erotic experience. Many girls are thwarted in their active attempts to find pleasure and love. Others try hard but make mistakes; some act in ways they later find regrettable or embarrassing or merely amusing. Many girls end up ambivalent and confused about just what they want. Some, of course, are luckier; they are able to stick to their dreams and find strategies for claiming what they need and desire, or craft new meanings for the erotic, and thereby resolve at least some of the conflict that sexual maturity creates. Different girls tread different paths across the terrain of sexuality and Eros.

Implications for Ethics

I argued in chapter 2 that feminist theologies of the erotic offer an insufficient basis for sexual ethics, for several reasons: They misconstrue how power works on the erotic, they substitute overconfident libertarian discourse about the erotic for sober reflection on how the erotic is constructed, they embrace a voluntaristic view of liberation, and they advocate a norm of relationality that is potentially counterproductive. Now we are in an even better position to justify these criticisms. Psychological and psychoanalytic theories have not only shed light on the empirical evidence gathered in chapter 4, but they have also helped us appreciate further the complexity of female erotic experience and the need to better theorize it.

We can now see that meanings of the erotic are linked to gender and power in subtle and indirect ways. Not only do authority figures frown upon girls' passionate expression and ignore girls' sexuality, though they do. Not only does society "teach" or "instill" in girls the idea that they should not display eroticism, though it does. Not only does the Christian religion denigrate the body and its passions, though this outlook may still prevail in certain areas. These repressive dynamics undoubtedly occur, but they cannot alone explain the magnetism of certain ideas about the erotic. Repression does not explain how people adopt certain patterns of behavior again and again, making them habitual, nor does religion account for the fact that certain meanings of the erotic become, as Jessica Benjamin puts it, "anchored in the hearts" of people.[64] People for whom society distorts their erotic experiences cling to the so-called distortions. Girls and women are not just influenced by others; girls subscribe to and embody certain constructions of the erotic. They do not just grow accustomed over time to thinking and acting in certain patterned ways; their own thoughts and actions help to reinforce and solidify those patterns. The experiences that feminist theologians of the erotic call inauthentic feel authentic enough to many girls and women; they wear them like a second skin. Sometimes girls and women even enjoy them. In other words, oppression does not only occur when institutions like society, family, and church forbid or restrain ideas and behaviors. Oppression does not only operate when "outside" forces like sexism, racism, and heterosexism bear down upon hapless individuals. As Foucault wrote:

> If power were never anything but repressive, if it never did anything but to say no, do you really think one would be brought to obey it? What makes power hold good, what makes it accepted, is simply the fact that it doesn't only weigh on us as a force that says no, but that it traverses and produces things, it induces pleasure, forms knowledge, produces discourse.[65]

Therefore, as Benjamin writes, "Only when we realize that power is not simply prohibition can we step outside the framework of choosing

---

64. Benjamin, *Bonds of Love*, 5. She explains the purpose of her work: "Above all, this book seeks to understand how domination is anchored in the hearts of the dominated."

65. Michel Foucault, "Truth and Power," in *Power/Knowledge: Selected Interviews and Other Writings*, ed. Colin Gordon (New York: Pantheon, 1980), 119.

between repressive authority and unbridled nature."[66] Feminist theologies of the erotic present us with such a choice because they accept this framework. They pit repressive authorities like religion, state, and patriarchy against the liberative force of the female erotic and claim that the latter would naturally flourish, unbridled, were it not for the former. They advocate a revolution against authority and a reclamation of women's natural erotic power. We are now in a position to understand that this framework is overly simplified and therefore a false choice. We know that the erotic is never "unbridled" but always saddled to complex dynamics of attachment and separation, recognition and assertion, relationality and independence. We also know that power traverses the formative relationships that provide girls and boys with their erotic knowledge, even at a very early age.

Raised in relationships that early on are marked by certain compromises, trade-offs, and preoccupations, many girls grow up thinking about themselves as erotic in ways that may be limited but are also compelling. Family structures that contain within them gendered power imbalances provide the scaffolding upon which daughters' erotic education is built. The meaning of the erotic for them will forever bear the imprint of those structures. Encouraging women to say "Yes" to the erotic thus provokes the question: Which form of the erotic would thereby be affirmed, and according to whose definition? The answer is not simply a matter of yes or no, but of which possibilities for the erotic can be created and who will be empowered to do the creative work. In short, while feminist theologies of the erotic are not necessarily wrong about the damage done to women by repressive authorities, they miss the constructive activity that keeps women reproducing those "damaging" patterns. This activity complicates the neat paradigm wherein impure patriarchy represses pure female nature. Somehow the ongoing reproduction of certain meanings of the erotic must be accounted for, which is what I have tried to do by theorizing the erotic.

Transformation will occur in the messy space where girls and women construct the erotic. We can now see why the power to liberate erotic patterns will never be the sole product of individuals as individuals. On her own, a woman cannot haul up the anchors in her heart. She cannot disentangle herself from the web of constructions that have been accumulating there since childhood. Women's erotic liberation must be a communal pro-

---

66. Benjamin, *Bonds of Love*, 4.

cess because the erotic is communally produced. Ultimately, the logic of
this chapter points in part to a broad dismantling of the gender inequal-
ities that structure contemporary American families; if Jessica Benjamin
and Nancy Chodorow are correct, the gender-structured family and its
pattern of exclusive female parenting is a significant factor in how the
erotic is built. Feminist theologians of the erotic do envision liberation
as a communal process of transformation. Our work fills in some of the
details of that vision.

We are not yet in a position to know what transformed experience will
look like, especially not in concrete terms. Since our understanding of
experience is and always will be mediated through the contexts that form
it, we cannot glean normative visions for the erotic directly from women's
present experiences. Many women may be "more relational" than men,
which may profoundly shape their eroticism; but if women do possess
this special quality, it does not necessarily merit reinforcing. As we learned
in this chapter, relationality is a mixed blessing conferred on women from
an early age. We ought to be dubious about reinforcing it, for excelling at
relationship can prevent women from developing the opposite but equally
necessary qualities of separation, self-assertion, and independence.

Finally, this chapter has demonstrated an alternative way of theorizing
the erotic to what we typically find in feminist theologies of the erotic. As
I argued in chapter 3, feminist theologies of the erotic are compromised
in three ways. Like other experiential feminisms, these theologies assume
that women's experience (a) has a common core, (b) interprets itself, and
(c) directly yields a normative vision. I avoid problem "a" by not assuming
that women's nature or women's oppression creates a core of experience
that is common to all women. First, in examining two different tendencies
that adolescent girls exhibit (distress and romantic obsession), I acknowledge at least some diversity of experience. I deliberately avoid claiming
that adolescence is the same for all girls. Feminist theologians of the erotic
are not always as careful and tend to imply that women all have the same
experiences by virtue of their being women.

Second, I do not assume the presence of one essential or ontological
thing called "the female erotic." Feminist theologies of the erotic posit
an erotic with a fixed nature. They further homogenize erotic experience
by assuming that the erotic is naturally good. At times, as in the case of
Brock's theology, they conflate psychological concepts with ontological
categories (e.g., the "relational self") and thus claim deeper essentialism

than is warranted. While I make many claims in this chapter about the commonality of girls' psychology and their experiences growing up, I do not make claims about girls' inherent nature or the erotic's inherent nature. Instead, I offer one line of reasoning, using psychological and psychoanalytic theories, for how the meaning of erotic experience is constructed in similar ways among girls. I submit that this approach is a different way of interpreting commonality of experience that highlights the contextuality of experience; assumes that any commonalities observed are historically specific and subject to change; and emphasizes social bonds between people, arguing that these bonds, not biology or nature, are what constitute identity. This form of interpretation is preferable because while it still has explanatory power, its claims remain provisional and open to revision given different contexts.

I avoid having to make the second claim — that women's experience interprets itself — by insisting that theory mediate experience. Were we to assume that what we hear in girls' speech exactly corresponds to some truth about their experience, we would have to conclude, for example, that girls' intelligence suffers during adolescence. We would have to assume either that they are not very smart or that adolescence automatically renders them confused and passive. In fact, we have seen that some early psychoanalytic theorists made such assumptions because they applied theories derived from boys' experience to girls. Feminist theologies of the erotic ironically run a parallel risk by assuming that women's experience speaks its own truth about the erotic — indeed, that women's experience corrects earlier theological assumptions about Eros. They assume that the power of the erotic working for good can be discerned directly from women's descriptions of their experience. Feminist theologies of the erotic would have us believe that the positive power of the erotic is the way things *really* are, but this condition would mean that erotic confusion, silence, and preoccupation become anomalies in girls' and women's experience. They do not fit the description of the erotic as working for good; therefore, they must be exceptions to the rule. The approach I am pursuing corrects this problem by assuming that experience is not transparent but needs some kind of interpretation before becoming revelatory. The same logic holds for claims about women's relationality. As Carol Gilligan herself has come to realize, if women's inclination toward relationship is simply taken at face value, one may fail to uncover crises in women's lives that precipitate it. By assuming not that the patterns one observes must represent "the way things are" but rather require explanation, one stays alert to the possibility that new light can be shed on old problems.

Third, in building a normative vision for sexual relationship, I depart from feminist theologies of the erotic by using experience indirectly rather than directly. Because they favor women's experience, feminist theologies of the erotic tend to assume a correspondence between experience and the divine or moral will. Sometimes their claims about the uniqueness of the female erotic are barely distinguishable from their claims about God. While I take a cue from insights about human relationship derived from observations of experience, I do not simply lift up one particular aspect of female experience as a moral norm, but rather I propose a norm for relationship that offers promise for relieving at least some of the misery many girls and women voice. The normative vision I propose is more pragmatic than visions grounded in transhistorical claims about reality. The vision is directed toward empowering people to cope with the inevitable ambiguities and tensions of erotic life and toward constructing trusting relationships that nurture rather than erode people's ability to flourish within them. To that project I now turn.

S I X

Establishing a Sexual Ethic
of Trust

Whatever matters to human beings, trust is the atmosphere in which it thrives.
— Sissela Bok, *Lying: Moral Choice in Public and Private Life*

I N THIS STUDY, I have argued that feminist theologies of the erotic embody a level of confidence in the power of Eros that is unwarranted by the complexity of erotic experience and the reality of many people's erotic lives. Many theologians seem content to set sexual ethics upon a foundation of renewed confidence in the erotic. They acknowledge that many sexually active people are troubled and confused, especially when attempting to make sense of gender, power, and sexuality. But theologians remain confident that by thinking differently about the erotic, we can resolve these difficulties. They continue to express faith in people's ability to imagine the erotic in new ways. I have argued, instead, against the idea that establishing the true meaning of sexuality can resolve its moral ambiguity, especially where adolescents are concerned. In this chapter, therefore, I suggest an alternate perspective from which to view the moral problems of adolescent sexuality (and, by implication, sexual ethics more generally): the perspective of trust. If the presumed goal of sexual morality can no longer be to figure out with precision the meaning and purpose of Eros, then the goal might instead be to secure enough trust between sexual partners to weather the ambiguity and vagary of erotic desiring.

Many theologians, especially those whom I have called feminist theologians of the erotic, continue to express faith in people's ability to imagine the erotic differently. Imaginative work, in fact, occupies a great deal of space within sexual ethics. Marvin Ellison, for example, writes:

Our socialization in a racist patriarchal culture frustrates our desire to be rightly connected, but — wonder of wonders — our imaginations help us envision alternative ways of loving beyond the limited roles the culture has assigned us.[1]

Ellison often calls his ethic of erotic justice a "mature" or "progressive" one, thereby contrasting his liberating, feminist, and sex-positive theology with earlier theologies of sex and gender. He, like others, believes that new ideology — rethinking and reimagining sex and love — will be what moves sexual ethics forward.

> Living comfortably with change and ambiguity requires maturity and a willingness to delight in difference and novelty. It also requires confidence in our collective ability to make meaningful moral distinctions and responsible choices. Religious communities should not be policing people's sex lives, but rather educating them about this real world of sexual diversity and expanding their moral imaginations.[2]

Perhaps some healthy skepticism regarding people's imaginative abilities would represent a genuinely mature ethic. Ideology critique alone cannot resolve all the moral ambiguities of sexual activity, especially where adolescents are concerned who are even less able than adults to reimagine their own experience. This study has shown that girls' perplexity about sex and love often results from contradictory constructions of femininity vying for their moral imagination. On a conscious level, girls attempt to be nurturing and sexy, nice and seductive, all at the same time. Unconsciously, they vacillate between the priorities of relationship and independence. Sometimes they try to conform to notions of femininity by disavowing themselves and some of their desires; sometimes they become obsessive in their desiring. Girls' failure to recognize, let alone resolve, the near impossibility of these contradictory constructions indicates less about the limits of their moral imagination than it does about the illogic of "feminine" adolescent sexuality with which they have to work.

In other words, cultural and psychological dynamics that limit the range of the imaginable affect even the faculty of moral imagination. The erotic

---

1. Marvin Ellison, *Erotic Justice: A Liberating Ethic of Sexuality* (Louisville, Ky.: Westminster/ John Knox Press, 1996), 83.

2. Ellison, *Erotic Justice,* 88.

is shaped at levels deeper than human consciousness can always access. Earlier chapters have sought to show how constructions of the erotic lodge inside girls' psyches, ultimately producing certain erotic behaviors. Girls' psychic processes that they themselves do not fully control often hamper the ability to imagine new ways of conducting themselves erotically and sexually. This condition obscures, rather than clears, the meaningfulness of moral distinctions and sexual choices. Given this situation, any individual girl's moral maturity may ultimately be a matter of good fortune; collectively, the moral fate of female adolescence depends on fundamental transformation in parenting, family structure, education, socialization, and gender relations as a whole.

Within the scope of this book, I have not been able to respond to all of the social, political, and economic factors affecting female adolescent sexuality, nor have I attempted to. But I am now in a position to address some of the moral questions that concern sexual ethicists and others who worry about adolescent sexual activity. While erotic experience includes more than sex, it is sexual activity that engenders the most moral concern. And so I turn now to considering the specific question of what adolescent girls need in order to make good choices about sexual relationships. When is a sexual relationship morally justified? After all, we should not assume that the pain of double standards and unsatisfactory consequences will stop adolescent girls from seeking pleasure and happiness in intimate relationships. Nor should it. Erotic satisfaction does not have to wait for the eschaton, or, as some feminists would say, until "after the revolution." While genuinely complex, painful, and frustrating, sexuality is also genuinely pleasurable and its pleasure justifiably sought. Moreover, even though gender roles and expectations remain unclear, times have changed *enough* to permit teenage girls unprecedented freedom in the sexual realm — and most of them would not wish to turn back the clock. While girls may value moral clarity, they also value the opportunity they now enjoy to grow and define themselves through various forms of romantic expression and erotic flourishing.

We know, in short, that adolescent girls will continue to engage in sexual activity that carries some risk of psychic and sometimes physical harm, and whose meaning is often difficult even for them to know. They are vulnerable to mixed messages about being female and having erotic feelings, and yet they must still make decisions about when to become sexually active and with whom. Under such conditions, the ethical challenge thus becomes one of making moral decisions in the midst of moral ambiguity. How is it possible to engage in a shared activity like sex when its moral meaning(s) remains unclear?

Ethicists seeking to offer a moral perspective on situations of ambiguity and vulnerability, where the moral actors nevertheless must move forward in some meaningful and responsible way, sometimes turn to the notion of trust. Interpersonal trust, viewed as something actively cultivated rather than simply assumed, can provide a safe context for moral choice when the precise meaning or *telos* of the chosen actions cannot be determined. Trust can sometimes lift the agonizing burden off of making choices. As one sociologist puts it, trust enables human beings to face the inevitable complexity and uncertainty of their lives while moving forward despite it. "The complexity of the future world is reduced by the act of trust."[3] With respect specifically to adolescent sexual behavior, the more a girl can trust herself and her partner, the better she will be able to tolerate the remaining ambiguity about the meaning of sex. If we can no longer presume that the moral ambiguity of girls' sexual lives will be resolved by their figuring out the "true" and proper meaning of erotic passion, and if we assume, furthermore, that the meanings of Eros and sex may continue to shift even throughout the rest of their lives, then the ethical task becomes one of reducing complexity as much as possible. One way to accomplish this task is to emphasize the importance of trust in sexual relationship.

The Nature of Trust

Philosopher Edmund Pellegrino writes that "trust is ineradicable in human relationships. Without it, we could not live in society or attain even the rudiments of a fulfilling life. Without trust, we could not anticipate the future and we would therefore be paralyzed into inaction."[4] Within human life in general and the moral life in particular, the need to trust others becomes necessary because we are historically situated beings who live out

3. Niklas Luhmann, *Trust and Power* (New York: John Wiley & Sons, 1979), 20.

4. Edmund D. Pellegrino, "Trust and Distrust in Professional Ethics," in *Ethics, Trust and the Professions: Philosophical and Cultural Aspects,* ed. Edmund D. Pellegrino, Robert M. Veatch, and John P. Langan (Washington, D.C.: Georgetown University Press, 1991), 69. As Pellegrino's statement makes clear, in this context we are primarily referring to trust as an action, rather than an attitude or sentiment. People make choices about when to trust and when to reserve it, and those choices make it possible to live in society and attain the rudiments of fulfillment.

our lives in time. Historicity enmeshes us in complexity and exposes us to chance. As we have seen in this study, for example, the family structures and friendship networks that people grow up in profoundly influence the texture of individuals' lives. Trust is one approach — others are planning and precaution — that people take to manage the challenge of having to live life out over time and its ever unfolding uncertainties.[5] In addition to historicity, human life is characterized by sociality. As social creatures, human beings constantly interact with other persons — and the myriad possibilities of their situations — adding even further complexity to the moral life. Again, trust serves to reduce the unpredictability of the human situation and brings a measure of stability to a life entwined with others'. Trust makes a life lived among others manageable. Sociologist Niklas Luhmann uses the image of pruning to describe what a decision to trust accomplishes: "The problem of trust therefore consists in the fact that the future contains far more possibilities than could ever be realized in the present. . . . [M]an must therefore prune the future so as to measure up with the present — i.e., reduce complexity."[6]

If it could be diagrammed, interpersonal trust would typically look something like an arrow with three points along it: Person A entrusts Person B with Valued Thing C.[7] In the act of entrusting, one person hands over to someone else something dear for the other to take care of. "Something dear" might mean anything from a treasured possession to secret information to one's own embodied, impassioned, confused self. In an erotic relationship, we might say that we entrust our sense of self to others. Whatever the case, in all trust relationships one person chooses to give to another for safekeeping something that matters. In choosing whom to trust, and with what, Person A gives some shape to her future, reducing the possibilities for what will happen to Valued Thing C. Person A also initiates a special relationship with Person B that binds them together and excludes others, at least as far as C is concerned. Trusters act

---

5. Margaret Farley makes a similar point about the human need to make commitments. Through them we bind ourselves to certain future courses of action, which limits our freedom but also assures our lives and our relationships consistency, continuity, and meaning. See *Personal Commitments: Beginning, Keeping, Changing* (San Francisco: Harper & Row Publishers, 1986), particularly chap. 2. The nature of trust here described shares affinities with the nature of commitment described by Farley.

6. Luhmann, *Trust and Power*, 13.

7. For this model of the trust relationship, I am indebted to Annette Baier, who analyses trust as a "three-place predicate." Annette Baier, *Moral Prejudices: Essays on Ethics* (Cambridge: Harvard University Press, 1994), 101.

as though they are actually pruning the alternatives for what will happen to Thing C, and thereby in effect do prune them, at least as far as the felt experience of complexity is concerned.

A few examples might serve to illustrate the paradigm. Trust describes the way an infant gives over a great deal of its life, health, and selfhood to its mother. A young child entrusts its emotional stability to its family. A student entrusts her comprehension of science to her teacher. A friend entrusts his secrets to his confidante. A lover entrusts her feelings to her beloved. A husband entrusts his emotional well-being to his wife. Sometimes, of course, the process is mutual: Both Person A and Person B reciprocally entrust each other with the same thing. Or, as is perhaps more often the case, they reciprocally trust one another, but with different things that matter to each of them respectively. In all these examples, people's lives are ordered by their act of trust, reducing myriad possibilities to a few. The infant does not relinquish itself peacefully to just anyone's care; the student does not take everyone's word to be the truth; husbands and wives do not randomly share themselves and their intimacies. All of these trusters place their faith in someone or something and, having done so, experience more security because they have reduced the likelihood of harm that might befall them.[8]

Or so they hope. After all, trust is itself a risky strategy. "Yet to trust and entrust is to become vulnerable and dependent on the good will and motivations of those we trust. Trust, ineradicable as it is, is also always problematic," Pellegrino goes on to say.[9] Unlike other approaches to reducing complexity — such as planning and calculating — trust includes risk because it involves embracing the unknown. Parents might divorce; the science teacher might start teaching philosophy instead; the beloved might undergo a change of heart. The possibility always exists that the ones we trust might leave us, act recklessly with our well-being, disregard what matters to us, or simply misjudge our desires. The risk of being harmed in some way, while not always made explicit, is built into the process of trusting. Trust is, after all, different from other forms of complexity reduction. Unlike using factual information alone (as in calculation), trust involves using a combination of facts, interpretations, past experience,

---

8. We should note that the infant does not make a conscious choice to trust; therefore, infant trust is a somewhat exceptional example. I include it to underscore the point that trust is something we learn from a very early age.

9. Pellegrino, "Trust and Distrust in Professional Ethics," 69.

hopes, and simple goodwill. A truster places her trust in something just beyond herself, typically another person. She acts just beyond the limits of her certainty. "Trust goes beyond the information it receives and risks defining the future. . . . In trusting, one engages in action *as though* there were only certain possibilities in the future."[10] What Luhmann is saying is that trust is always a wager and, as such, inevitably involves some degree of artifice: When we trust, we act as if the world will remain the way we hope, and as if others will behave predictably, though we can never know for sure. As Luhmann puts it, "Trust always extrapolates from the available knowledge; it is . . . a blending of knowledge and ignorance."[11]

Nevertheless, trust becomes an action or strategy upon which human beings vitally depend, and choose both consciously and unconsciously, out of their desire to thrive. Trust is one of the vehicles in human life that supports and, indeed, renders possible human flourishing by making room for actions and relationships that would otherwise simply be too threatening. While inevitable risk resides in trusting, moral agents undertake it again and again in different circumstances about different decisions, because of its potential to open the door to future fulfillment and to bring them happiness.

Trust is important to erotic relationships, for people seek to flourish through such relationships and yet do not find their erotic flourishing guaranteed simply by being in one. As we have seen in this study, erotic relationships expose us to a wide range of human vulnerabilities, as do intense and intimate relationships of any kind. In particular, erotic partners become exposed to their own and the other's conscious and unconscious claims to self-assertion and union, to separation and attachment, and to all the behaviors deployed by the psyche to satisfy those claims. Erotic relationships bring into full relief all the psychic distress of two individuals' developmental struggles. Erotic relationships also tend to exacerbate, in often peculiar ways, the temptation to disavow either self or other. Added to these psychological risks, of course, is the problem that partners in erotic relationship often desire different things from the relationship. They entrust each other with different erotic desires and frequently need to find a way to balance them. Particularly when partners subscribe to different meanings for what is erotically satisfying, significant tension and

---

10. Luhmann, *Trust and Power,* 20 (emphasis added).
11. Luhmann, *Trust and Power,* 26.

risk of exacerbating vulnerability can arise simply because their respective ways of finding fulfillment and well-being conflict. In short, people seek erotic relationships because they address deep and basic yearnings for intimacy, pleasure, closeness, excitement, and power; yet those very yearnings also open them to vulnerability. The pleasure of Eros always treads closely to its danger.

Testing the Waters of Trust

Precisely because they require both risk and artifice, not all trust relationships are warranted. Sometimes to trust is to be foolhardy, flagrantly disregarding the reality of the historical and social situation. These characteristics may especially hold true in erotic relationships. Moreover, like the erotic, trust itself is elusive and impossible to extract, growing by implicit, rather than explicit, movement. By definition, the terms of trust cannot be spelled out ahead of time. Trust cannot be willed, stipulated in advance, or enforced. If it could, it would not be *trust,* but something else, like a negotiation or a contract. For these reasons, placing one's trust in others is not always wise; placing trust sometimes may be morally wrong.

Annette Baier is a feminist philosopher who has given extensive attention to the notion of trust and, more specifically, to the moral implications of trust relationships. As she puts it, either "proper" or "improper" trust is at work. Sometimes trust is warranted and sometimes it is not. As a feminist, Baier has often chosen to concentrate on relationships between men and women as paradigmatic of the need for trust. She brings the concept of power to bear upon the concept of trust, for she identifies vulnerability as the human condition that makes trust necessary.

Baier believes that trust is essentially accepted vulnerability. She concurs with the philosophers mentioned thus far that trusting is a risky act involving acknowledgment of one's vulnerability — to chance and to the power others may choose to exercise. But the truster accepts this vulnerability and places his trust in another. The crucial factor is accepting one's vulnerability willingly and honestly, not simply making an unthinking acquiescence. Baier has suggested, therefore, that the way to discern whether trust is proper is to test whether it "survives consciousness." This test may at first appear highly ironic, because we are so used to thinking of trust as an unconscious thing. But what Baier actually says is that the vulnerability associated with trusting should survive consciousness.

Usually people know how an invitation to trust initially makes them feel, whether the emotion is dread or apprehension or relief. Sometimes they can explicitly identify the aspect of the invitation that makes them feel the way they do. Perhaps the personality of the other person or the height of the stakes involved is the causative factor. To the extent that people are able to name what makes them vulnerable when they begin to trust, Baier says, trust is sound. Trust is proper when its vulnerabilities can be exposed. The truster goes in with her eyes open, so to speak. She can identify what she is specifically relying on in the other as she places her trust. In addition, she can risk telling her feelings to the one she is considering trusting. Good trust survives the truster's admission of vulnerability. If the truster cannot, for some reason, name the feature that makes her willing to trust, she should not do so.

> To the extent that what the truster relies on for the continuance of the trust relation is something which, once realized by the trusted, is likely to lead to (increased) abuse of trust and eventually to destabilization and destruction of that relation, the trust is morally corrupt.[12]

The "survival test" applies both to trusting and being entrusted. In other words, the trusted must be able, insofar as possible, to name the vulnerability, to be free to warn the truster when not to trust. This statement is the test's second condition. When B knows that A is overrelying on something, B must be able to say so. Only insofar as the trusted can accept or reject the vulnerability of being entrusted (in other words, insofar as they can beg out of a trust offer) is the trust sound.

Baier summarizes her test by saying that two conditions are constitutive of morally proper trust: that it can withstand being made explicit, and that the trusted person has been given a chance to withdraw. "Plausible conditions for proper trust will be that it survives consciousness, by both parties, and that the trusted has had some opportunity to signify acceptance or rejection, to warn the trusting if their trust is inappropriate."[13] Baier argues that when both conditions are met, a choice to trust is morally sound because both truster and trusted are aware of what is at stake for the other, and both have reason to honor those stakes. Exposing

---

12. Baier, *Moral Prejudices*, 123.
13. Baier, *Moral Prejudices*, 99.

the accepted vulnerability reveals the "soft spots" in the trust relationship, as it were, and a relationship that nevertheless survives must be legitimate.

Consider three examples, one of proper trust and two where trust is improper. (They are taken from outside the realm of erotic relationship.) If I entrust you with a secret, what I am likely relying on is your ability to keep secrets. If I have no reason to fear or hesitate telling you that I am relying on your secret-keeping ability, then my trust in you is probably sound. If you can tell me that, in fact, you are either lousy or very good at keeping secrets, then our trust relationship is almost surely a good one. Under these circumstances, entrusting you with my secret, should I so decide, and you accepting my trust are appropriate.[14] Note that testing the soundness of trust is not the same as predicting its success. Circumstances may arise that compel you to spill the secret after all, despite your initial assurances. In this case, I will not have succeeded in safeguarding the secret that I value. But that result does not necessarily mean that I was wrong to trust you. My trust may still have been appropriate. Trusting you again in the future may even be proper.

If, on the other hand, I entrust you with secret information because I know you lack the intelligence to understand it and would be too embarrassed to admit so, I am relying instead on your stupidity and your pride. Probably I cannot tell you that I am relying on your stupidity, so therefore my trust is unfair. You cannot refuse to keep secret the information because you are embarrassed to admit to not understanding it. I have, in effect, coerced you into accepting my trust by keeping its conditions secret. In this example, I may appear to be "trusting" you and that you are letting yourself be entrusted, but the trust relationship is tainted. Its moral footing is insecure because neither one of us can be explicit about the conditions underlying the trust. The situation makes us both vulnerable (you perhaps more than me), but neither of us can name the vulnerability. We cannot talk about it. In short, in this example my "trust" is a mere seizing of power that is morally improper.

As for a third example, let us say that after a period of hesitation, I decide to entrust you with secret information about my past because you have finally made me feel too guilty for not sharing it. After telling you the information, all I can rely on for keeping it a secret is your smugness. And

---

14. This example tests only the propriety of the trust. It abstains from questioning the morality of the secret itself (i.e., whether my concealing the information is proper or whether I am spilling a "guilty secret").

yet I scarcely want to call you smug, for fear of further alienating you. In this case, you have coerced my trust. You exploited my vulnerability. And yet if you gloat too much over my finally having shared my past with you, I will become disinclined to trust you with any more information. You will have ruined the "trust" between us.

In the second and third examples, the trust is rotten, and even calling it "trust" is inaccurate. One of the primary ways we can tell that trust is wrong in these cases is that the vulnerability that each party accepts cannot be revealed. Either the truster or the trusted suffers undue vulnerability — an abuse of trust. The trust is both flimsy and improper because in order to sustain it, someone has to rely on artifice or guile.

Baier offers her own examples of morally corrupt trust relationships: ones that survive by virtue of the truster's gullibility, ones where the trusted is skilled at covering up breaches in their trustworthiness, ones where either truster or trusted is able to charm the other into forgiving past breaches of trust. Gullibility, guile, and charm are the sorts of qualities relied on that, once revealed, tend to destabilize trust relationships. Ignorance and fear also generally serve to destabilize trust, once they come to light as factors in its establishment or maintenance. (Baier points out, however, that ignorance and fear do not always destabilize trust, as when fear of crime motivates the general public to rely on the police to stop it.)[15]

Baier phrases her trust test a second way: "A trust relationship is morally bad to the extent that either party relies on qualities in the other which would be weakened by the knowledge that the other relies on them."[16] In other words, trust relationships are constructed out of expectations and assumptions, such as personal qualities, gifts, or shared ends, on which the partners mutually rely. Some of these expectations are less sound than others. When they are exposed, human nature tends to ensure that the trust relationship will grow weaker. None of us ultimately wants to be merely flattered into a trust relationship. "The knowledge that others are counting on one's nonreciprocated generosity or good nature or forgiveness can have the power of the negative, can destroy trust."[17] On the other hand, the power of the positive can strengthen trust: once I know the good qualities my partner is relying on in me, I will likely rise to the occasion of his trust.

---

15. Baier, *Moral Prejudices*, 124.
16. Baier, *Moral Prejudices*, 123.
17. Baier, *Moral Prejudices*, 124.

Where each relies on the other's love, concern for some common good, or professional pride in competent discharge of responsibility, knowledge of what the other is relying on in one need not undermine but will more likely strengthen those relied-on features. They survive exposure as what others rely on in one in a way that some forms of stupidity, fear, blindness, ignorance, and gullibility normally do not.[18]

Assuming normal self-esteem, most people are either pleased or daunted by receiving another's trust (and assuming mutual goodwill, are free to accept or refuse — Baier's second condition). Exposing the implicit expectations and assumptions underlying the trust is therefore an effective test of whether the trust is wise.

Baier's test is not perfect, nor would it suffice as a sole basis for sexual ethics. One might note, for instance, that the test is open to false positives, which Baier herself admits. In other words, she acknowledges that people sometimes found their trust on morally questionable bases that are not necessarily weakened upon exposure. In fact, Baier specifically mentions sexual relationships in this regard. She cites the example of a predilection for sexual bondage. If A confesses to B that she likes being a slave and wants B to be her master, this confession may only encourage B's aggression and hostility.

There are other mental states whose sensitivity to exposure as relied on by others seems more variable: good nature, detachment, inattention, generosity, forgivingness, and sexual bondage to the other party may not be weakened by knowledge that others count on their presence in one to sustain some wanted relationship, especially if they are found equally in both parties.[19]

One might also note that in addition to the problem of false positives, Baier's test is problematic because it does not in itself discourage people from building trust relationships on overly narrow, trite, and possibly even harmful expectations. The test simply affirms that so long as each other's trustworthy qualities can be openly sustained, trusting is sound. In its agnosticism regarding the qualities relied upon, the test approves both profound and shallow relationships alike. While it may serve to identify

18. Baier, *Moral Prejudices*, 123–24.
19. Baier, *Moral Prejudices*, 124.

trustworthiness, the test ironically does not evaluate which qualities are worth trusting. Applied to erotic relationships, Baier's test does not necessarily screen out relationships of sexual bondage, as the above passage indicates. The test does not, in and of itself, favor relationships where partners love each other and pledge permanence — qualities that many people believe to be important for sexual relationships.

Happily, we need not choose only one moral norm for sexual ethics. Trust is but one norm among many that should be applied to sexual relationships. We could upon reflection decide, for example, that while love and permanence may not be required to establish trust, they certainly help. Perhaps even the most trust-filled sexual relationships are ones developed over time by people who love each other. We could also remind ourselves that trust is like a habit which, when practiced long and hard enough, sustains human flourishing and thereby promotes new growth. In other words, while working to establish a mutually trusting relationship, sexual partners will likely come to discover and even trust further qualities in each other and ends they share.

Finally, some people might respond to Baier's test that she has simply made the act of trusting entirely more complicated than it needs to be. We should simply avoid trusting scoundrels. Yet such a simple outlook would miss the points made earlier about trust. Often we really need to trust others despite poor circumstances, or we choose to trust in order to expedite matters or maintain relationships we cherish. We do not wait for ideal circumstances but risk trusting because we desire to flourish and secure things that will contribute to our flourishing.

Trust Versus Distrust

Sometimes when the stakes are high but people still need or want to entrust themselves to another, they choose a different but related strategy: friendly distrust. Distrust, as I am using the term, is not necessarily the opposite of trust or the absence of it. Distrust instead describes a different relational choice that still allows two people to act in concert but with more safeguards erected around their relationship. In relationships of friendly distrust, partners acknowledge the ambiguities of their situation and realize that neither may know the full meaning of what they seek to achieve from it. Distrust represents a more skeptical, conservative, slightly more distant stance vis-à-vis the other party but a stance that still makes room for entrusting and seeking fulfillment.

To gain further perspective on the difference between trust and distrust, and on the question of their advisability within erotic relationship, let us first consider briefly a radically different kind of relationship, yet one in which many of the same issues arise. I have in mind the professional relationship between a client and a practitioner. In looking at trust and distrust within a professional relationship, I do not mean to suggest in any way that adolescent girls are like clients and their boyfriends like professionals. Rather, I am suggesting that professional relationships are similar to erotic relationships because in both trust between the parties is commonly considered very important and equally elusive.[20] In both types of relationship, the parties seek to meet basic needs of human flourishing but do not know just what will ensure it. Some level of trust in each other is crucial, and yet trusting is risky given the uncertainties of the situation.

Not unlike ethicists interested in sexual matters, many ethicists addressing the professions rue the paucity of relationships between professionals and clients that display genuine trust. Frequently ethicists respond with offers of ways that trust might be restored.[21] Others simply concede the decline of professional-client trust and look instead for ways clients can protect themselves against breaches of trust suffered at the hands of professionals.[22] Underlying this difference in perspective are basic questions about the nature of trust relationships. As Pellegrino, Veatch, and Langan ask in the preface to their book *Ethics, Trust, and the Professions,* "Are the relationships with patients or clients to be understood as contractual, covenantal, or commodity transactions?"[23] Different answers to this question produce different ethics.

Why is trust between client and professional assumed to be so critical in the first place? Interestingly enough, one reason points to a similarity between sexual and professional-client relationships. As Pellegrino says, the vulnerability experienced by clients in large part generates their need

20. See Pellegrino, Veatch, and Langan, *Ethics, Trust, and the Professions,* especially essays by Sokolowski and Zaner on the fiduciary relationship, Buchanan and Brock on trust and professional knowledge, and Meilaender on professional virtues.

21. One empirical example of attempts at restoring trust in professionals is the proliferation of workshops and seminars in the workplace through training. Professional schools also seek to prevent professional misconduct through education.

22. An example, to counter the one above, is the proliferation of law firms specializing in malpractice suits.

23. Pellegrino, Veatch, and Langan, *Ethics, Trust, and the Professions,* viii.

to trust professionals. And as he suggests, the need for trust increases with the need for assistance.

> Trust is most problematic when we are in states of special dependency — in illness, old age, or infancy, or when we are in need of healing, justice, spiritual help, or learning. This is the situation in our relationships with the professions whom circumstances force us to trust. We are forced to trust professionals, if we wish access to their knowledge and skill. We need the help of doctors, lawyers, ministers, or teachers to surmount or cope with our most pressing human needs. We must depend on their fidelity to trust and their desire to protect, rather than to exploit, our vulnerability.[24]

In particular, the bewilderment and uncertainty that come with needing to ask for help characterize clients' vulnerability before professionals. By definition, patients, defendants, parishioners, students, and other "clients" find themselves in situations whose meanings they cannot entirely fathom. If they could, they would not need the professional help they have sought. Medical patients, for example, are frequently ignorant of or perplexed by the changes in their bodies that signal illness. They cannot understand these changes, let alone treat them, on their own. Richard Zaner identifies the phenomenology of being a patient as an experience of uncertainty:

> The sick person concretely experiences his/her body as a source of uncertainty: for instance, what is causing pain, how long it will last, what it signifies now and for the future. . . . Illness itself is alienating, rupturing the person's usual ways of feeling, acting, moving, and integrating body and self. Indeed, a crucial dimension of trust — trust in one's own body — is existentially breached, the person's bodily experiences taking on a kind of inner strangeness — new and peculiar feelings in one's body, for example, that are often at best difficult to convey.[25]

Patients enter into relationships with doctors out of a desire to make themselves whole again. They place their bodies (often literally) in the hands of doctors. Since, by definition, patients lack the expertise to judge with specificity what kind of help and healing they desire, they accept

---

24. Pellegrino, "Trust and Distrust in Professional Ethics," 69.
25. Richard M. Zaner, "Trust and the Patient-Physician Relationship," in Pellegrino, Veatch, and Langan, *Ethics, Trust, and the Professions*, 50–51.

a degree of not knowing and simply absorb that risk, which is why the
doctor-patient relationship is sometimes seen as paradigmatic of trust:
The patient entrusts her well-being to another to seek the good of health.
Robert Sokolowski describes it this way:

> [T]he professional deals not only with my possessions but with me.
> If I go to a mechanic or to a dry cleaner, even one that provides "pro-
> fessional dry cleaning," I hand over my car or my jacket to someone
> else, but in dealing with a doctor or a lawyer or a teacher, I sub-
> mit myself to be determined in my future condition by the one I
> consult. . . . [26]

Sokolowski is one ethicist who concludes that trust is indispensable to
the professional-client relationship. He would say that clients are forever
vulnerable, in need of assistance, and facing situations where they must
entrust themselves to professionals. Professionals, on the other hand, always have something — knowledge, skills, or services — that clients need,
and therefore always have a degree of power and authority over clients.
Trust bridges this gap. Trustworthiness in professionals is what eases the
tension clients feel in being vulnerable and powerless. The only problem,
as he sees it, is to find ways to minimize for clients the risks associated
with trusting. Edmund Pellegrino concurs:

> Given the empirical inevitability of trust in professional relation-
> ships, what is needed are not attempts to eradicate it, but rather a
> reconstruction of professional ethics grounded in its ineradicabil-
> ity. Such an ethic of trust must be based in the "internal morality"
> of each profession — those ethical obligations that arise in the na-
> ture of each profession, the kind of human activity each profession
> encompasses. [27]

Some of the "ethical obligations" that Pellegrino, Sokolowski, and
others cite include the professional's obligation to be conscientious, to discern the client's best interest, and to respect client autonomy. Professionals,
according to this line of thinking, are obliged to share as much information as they can with their clients, doing so in a way that their clients
can understand. They must not assume that their clients share their own

---

26. Robert Sokolowski, "The Fiduciary Relationship and the Nature of Professions," in
Pellegrino, Veatch, and Langan, *Ethics, Trust, and the Professions,* 28.
27. Pellegrino, "Trust and Distrust in Professional Ethics," 76.

beliefs and values but must try to see the case from their clients' points of view. If their clients make decisions that contradict what they would have decided, client decisions ought generally to be respected.[28] A professional's character also becomes important. What clients rely on in their relationships with professionals are the professionals' qualities of truthfulness, sensitivity, and caring concern. Therefore, professionals ought to work at developing these qualities if they want to be known as trustworthy.[29]

People who view trust as indispensable to the professional-client relationship tend to define that relationship in terms of a covenant. They argue that clients' relationship to professionals ought to be intimate in nature and based on care and compassion.[30] Such a high view of professional relationships can be countered by the sober realization that client trust may simply reinforce professional paternalism, an outdated concept that can be justified less frequently within professional practice. Familiar, intimate, and highly trusting relationships between, say, patients and their doctors belonged to an era when patient autonomy was less highly valued and doctors were more typically presumed to "know best." Now that patients and other types of clients enjoy more power, some would argue, a paternalistic professional-client relationship is inappropriate. Clients can and should expect to be treated more as equals of the professionals they engage and even as consumers of the services professional provide.

Philosophical reasons are also given for clients placing less trust in professionals. Robert Veatch, for example, argues that professionals are not, and never have been, all-knowing. Instead, their understanding of client well-being is actually highly constructed by their role as "experts." Their view of what constitutes well-being may even be narrow and inaccurate, rendering them actually somewhat untrustworthy. "It may be,"

---

28. Pellegrino believes, however, that professionals may also make decisions that deserve respect. He argues that professionals may rightfully refuse to provide certain services, such as abortions, on moral grounds. "Professional Neutrality: An Ethical Impossibility," keynote address for the Ninth Annual Meeting of the Association for Practical and Professional Ethics, February 27, 2000.

29. In addition to Meilaender's essay cited above, see, for example, David Luban, ed., *The Good Lawyer: Lawyers' Roles and Lawyers' Ethics* (Totowa, N.J.: Rowman and Allanheld, 1984), including Andreas Eshete, "Does a Lawyer's Character Matter?"; William F. May, "Professional Ethics: Setting, Terrain, and Teacher," in *Ethics Teaching in Higher Education,* ed. Daniel Callahan and Sissela Bok (New York: Plenum, 1980); and Bernard Williams, "Politics and Moral Character" in *Public and Private Morality,* ed. Stuart Hampshire (New York: Cambridge University Press, 1978).

30. See especially William F. May, *The Physician's Covenant: Images of the Healer in Medical Ethics* (Philadelphia: Westminster Press, 1983).

he writes, "that the very concept of trusting a professional is not a co-herent one."[31] Veatch means that professionals are by definition people who have achieved significant levels of education, training, and expertise. Professionals become professionals by devoting several years of their lives to learning a body of conceptual information and perfecting a repertoire of skills. Thus by definition they develop highly specialized subspheres of knowledge and interest. Clients value this perspective because they them-selves benefit from it. And yet, the very fact that professionals' knowledge is limited to such particular subspheres ironically distances them from clients. Specialization renders it more difficult for them to know their clients' total best interest.

> Once again, the problem is not that professionals are unworthy of trust because of their biases, lack of commitment, or lack of objectiv-ity. Even the most skilled, knowledgeable, and unbiased professional must constantly make evaluative and conceptual choices that must get incorporated into the presentation to the client. The lawyer's summary of the legal history, the teacher's selection of a syllabus of the important literature, and the accountant's choice of an ac-counting method all cloud the most impeccably devoted, skilled, and unbiased professional's presentations. Professionals cannot be trusted to present the facts objectively, not because of their short-comings as professionals, but because of the inherent limits in the process of reporting professional knowledge.[32]

In other words, though they possess great knowledge about some things, professionals do not know — and cannot be expected to know — everything their clients may hope they know. They may not be able to promote their clients' overall well-being because many aspects of it lie outside their area of expertise. "There is increasing reason to hold that modern professionals ought not to be able to know what the client's in-terests really are," Veatch says.[33] According to Veatch's logic, professionals are necessarily "untrustworthy" because of their high degree of special-ized knowledge and their inevitable commitment to ways of sharing that knowledge that may or may not always match their clients' needs and in-

---

31. Robert M. Veatch, "Is Trust of Professionals a Coherent Concept?" in Pellegrino, Veatch, and Langan, *Ethics, Trust, and the Professions,* 159.
32. Veatch, "Is Trust of Professionals a Coherent Concept?" 165–66.
33. Veatch, "Is Trust of Professionals a Coherent Concept?" 161.

terests. And if professionals cannot know their clients' best interest, can they serve it? Should they be entrusted with it?

Distrust As an Appropriate Stance

If professionals cannot be "trusted" to know and serve their clients' best interest, Veatch goes on to argue, distrust may be more appropriate. He believes that professionals should be committed to serving their clients and should admit and explain the values according to which they present facts and provide services. Beyond this, they should confess their fallibility and bias. One way of explaining Veatch's recommendation is that he thinks professionals ought to acknowledge the inevitable discrepancy between their way of viewing the world and what may be their clients'. Professionals and clients could mutually and openly acknowledge, rather than try to correct, the inherent asymmetry between what each knows and values. They could accept and embrace their different positions within the relationship. In other words, they could attempt to name, rather than obscure, the different meanings they ascribe to the very illness, need, or condition that brings them together.

One could call this a version of friendly distrust within the professional-client relationship. Distrust does not necessarily mean mistrust, that is, outright suspicion of harm or utter lack of confidence in the other. Rather distrust would be a form of relationship characterized by minimalism — in the degree of personalism, in intimacy, and especially of assumptions about commonly shared knowledge. Distrust assumes a minimal overlap between the meanings each partner ascribes to the situation. Distrust acknowledges the limitations on ever knowing completely the other's interests or the full extent of the concerns brought to the relationship, assuming that a trusting relationship will probably not come naturally or easily because of these obscured issues.

What are the advantages and disadvantages of trust and distrust, given this description of their difference? Certain advantages come with the latter. Distrust entails less risk for clients than trusting does. Adopting an attitude of distrust, rather than complete trust, moreover, prompts clients to learn as much as they can about their own problems. Less artifice exists in the relationship because a fully trusting demeanor need not be maintained. In fact, if clients were to accept that the professionals they consult are both fallible and biased toward the services they provided, clients might be empowered to investigate those services more thoroughly and not take them for granted. Clients might be forced to see that professionals do not automatically share their values, and, as a result, clients might also be encouraged to identify and state their own values more precisely. Within such an ethos, clients would be encouraged to exercise greater autonomy, to make their own decisions. Both client and professional would accept the contingency of their relationship and would not place excessive faith in it. Distrustful clients would actually experience more reassurance by taking less "on faith," if you will, and relying more on the stated premises of the relationship. Were distrust to force the terms of relationship out in the open, clients might actually feel they had more freedom and security.

Of course, distrust carries disadvantages as well. When less is risked, less is available to be gained. Distrustful relationships are circumscribed in what they can accomplish. A distrustful spirit of minimalism could lead clients to lower their desires, expectations, and dreams and could invite feelings of *caveat emptor.* An ethos of distrust might also encourage clients to view professionals as mere instruments of their desires. As for professionals, because distrust limits their discretionary power, they might feel that their commitment and creativity were hampered and therefore become tempted to regard their clients as a series of "cases" rather than unique individuals. Distrust might even lead to legalism and an excessive sense of self-protectiveness on either side of the relationship. In short, distrust could degenerate into mistrust.

In relationships where trust flourishes, by contrast, caring and concern could expand because both client and professional would enjoy a certain latitude in the way they relate to each other. Risking depth in their relationship might open up possibilities for each. An ethos of trust might allow the relationship to become close and personal in a way that could never be achieved under an ethos of distrust. If client and professional felt they knew one another, they might feel their efforts were synchronized and that they were more committed to their shared purpose.

The relevance of our discussion of professional relationship to erotic relationship should start by now to be apparent. We have identified uncertainty and vulnerability as common denominators of the two kinds of relationship. Like clients, lovers do not know exactly what the erotic feelings they experience mean and may very well bring different understandings of the relationship to it. I have previously argued that adolescent girls, in particular, are often anxious about the meaning of erotic passion and assume that relationships mean something quite specific without making this clear. Even when one person's feelings are clear, moreover, the other person may not share these feelings. And yet, not unlike clients, lovers want to enter erotic relationship because they want the fulfillment only it can bring.

Accordingly, the difficulty of trying to forge a satisfying and wholesome erotic relationship might be met in one of two ways: Erotic partners could adopt a stance of trust or, alternatively, one of distrust. They could open themselves fully, giving discretion to their partners and assuming shared purpose and mutual closeness. Or, they could take less for granted and lower both the stakes and the guarantees of the relationship. While I have presented these two strategies as contrasting choices, in truth most trust relationships likely fall somewhere along a spectrum between them. As in professional-client relationships, adolescents in love probably vacillate between distrust and trust, which is probably fitting.

Adolescent Sexuality and an Ethic of Trust

Bringing these reflections to bear directly on adolescent sexual relationships, we would conclude from the above discussion that an ethos of trust in sexual relationships would heighten the vulnerability they already experience and might increase the possibility that they will disavow themselves, while an ethos of distrust would protect them more even if it were to change their ideal aims. Let us recall for a moment the narratives we have heard from adolescent girls about sex, love, and romance. Take, for example, Sheila, whom Lori Stern interviewed in her study of female adolescent self-disavowal. Sheila offered a vivid image of two people standing silent in a sinking boat, each refusing to say anything to the other for fear of calling attention to their danger. As they stand trapped by their mutual hesitation, the boat slowly sinks. Sheila used this metaphor to confess to Stern her reluctance to tell her boyfriend that she wanted to end their sexual relationship. She knew her silence accomplished nothing, and even potentially endangered her, but she maintained it anyway. To repeat Sheila's words:

> It is like two people standing on a boat that they both know is sinking. I don't want to say anything to you because it will upset you, and you don't want to say anything to me because it will upset you.

And we are both standing here in water up to our ankles watching
it rise and I don't want to say anything to you.[34]

Sheila has, in effect, described a relationship of improper trust. She
could not entrust her boyfriend with the truth of why she did not want
to sleep with him. He, in turn, not only avoided discussing their relationship because doing so upset him, but he also urgently wanted sex and
was persuasive in getting it. Sheila was probably correct in her appraisal
that he could neither honestly participate in nor openly refuse the conversation about sex she wished to have. Therefore she could not trust him.
What Sheila attempted to do was resolve this impossible situation, at least
temporarily, by *pretending* to trust her boyfriend (which she voiced as pretending not to notice the water around her ankles). However, she knew
that the cost was disavowing herself, and that in the long run she could
not preserve both her own integrity and the relationship at the same time.
In effect, Sheila knew that the situation was untenable because the "trust"
between them was rotten, as her metaphor reveals. Their trust leaked as
badly as a sinking boat.

Let us also recall girls like Tracy and Nikki who seem to live almost entirely for romantic relationship — the ones who sleep in makeup,
drink from their boyfriends' coffee cups, let daydreams constantly distract
them, or drop out of school. These girls, as we recall, talk about little
else besides relationship and seem to rest their sense of identity almost
solely on whether they are romantically attached. They place high priority on the supposed fulfillment of being in relationship. We might say
that they entrust themselves to romance. Can this kind of trust survive
consciousness?

Sharon Thompson persuasively argues that many adolescent girls,
whether they acknowledge it or not, maintain the hope that their adolescent relationships might lead to love and marriage. Often even by their
own admission, many girls are on a "quest" for the perfect romance, as one
girl admitted when she said, "I want the ideal relationship." With some
girls, marriage found its way into nearly every conversation Thompson
had with them about their life goals. Can they tell their boyfriends this?

Girls today generally know that they cannot. Most know, at some level,
that the quest is an ideal attractive to them but unacceptable to their

---

34. Stern, "Disavowing the Self," 111.

male peers. Let us assume for a moment that some girls might be willing and able to make their expectations of true love and marriage clear, and find boyfriends willing and able to accept this expectation. In such cases, according to Baier's test, their trust would be proper, and the relationships they build unlikely to cause them harm. However much some of us as feminists might consider the goal of fairy-tale romance to be trivial and foolish, if the risk of hoping for it can be openly waged, who are we to judge? In some contexts, playing the game of romance by the rules of true love is fitting and fine. In reality, however, few girls today who hope that sexual involvement will secure the one true love of their dreams are positioned to state their desires so frankly, as previous chapters have shown. Their wish barely surfaces to consciousness. When girls finally become aware of their own logic, many of them reject it. They become aware that sexual involvement is often a game stacked against them from the start. The popular poem cited earlier expresses this dawning awareness: "When I met you, I liked you. / When I liked you, I loved you. / When I loved you, I let you. / When I let you, I lost you." Girls also start to perceive the gendered nature of the sexual game: Boys are usually playing by a different logic, and their rules usually prevail.

Many boys still take advantage of girls' vulnerability. They rely on the fact that girls are looking for love and promise to reciprocate that love in exchange for sex. In effect, they coerce girls' trust. Like our example of entrusting someone with secret information when made to feel guilty otherwise, girls feel they cannot refuse the invitation to trust or else they risk being cut off from relationship. The main thing they rely on is boys' desire for sex, and even they often accurately sense this desire to be transferable and hence fickle and flimsy. To the extent that girls cannot expose their reliance, for fear of losing love, they trust improperly. They know they cannot say: "Because I love you and want you to love me, I will let you have sex with me," even if they still harbor that fantasy privately. They become the compliant trusters. Caught in this trap, as I have already argued, girls become powerless relative to boys. Under these circumstances, relationships of trust are inappropriate because they exacerbate girls' vulnerability and powerlessness.

To be fair, sometimes girls know precisely what they are doing when they "trust" boys' promises of love. To the extent that they maintain the fantasy of true love knowing full well that it is a fantasy, their trust coerces their boyfriends, resting on an artifice of playing a game while pretending not to. To be additionally fair, many boys do not intend to be coercive. They may promise love genuinely thinking that they will fall in love.

In contrast to all these stories, however, some adolescent girls have rejected the logic of true love. In other words, some girls realize the fool-hardiness of entrusting adolescent sexual partners with their well-being and happiness. They adopt instead a stance of friendly distrust within their erotic relationships. They work at knowing their feelings, they are aware of their own vulnerability, and they keep their expectations of erotic rela-tionship to a minimum. We have not heard from such girls in this study, but their voices are real. Let us consider, for example, Anja, who was one of Thompson's interviewees. Thompson had asked her to describe a memory of sexual desire, and Anja chose to tell a story about flirting with a boy at a rock concert. Although the experience was very nice (and evi-dently quite memorable), the encounter led to nothing more than holding hands. They did not even look at each other. Their hands just found each other's.

> And it was really funny. It was really nice. And then the concert ended and the crowd started to disperse and I sort of looked at him. And I just couldn't bring myself to say anything to him, because I thought, No matter what I say, it'll just like shatter it, you know. So we kind of just let go of each other's hands and walked away.[35]

Anja sensed that this episode was complete and would not lead to a full-blown sexual relationship. She realized that she did not even want it to. She was content to leave it as a minimal encounter.

Later, Thompson asked Anja to describe "her first time" with her boy-friend, Monty. By the time she had sexual intercourse with Monty, Anja was certain of what she wanted, for she had been willing to wait until she felt a sense of certainty. When she finally decided to have sex, her decision was based primarily on her own feelings of desire as well as other reasons she was able to list.

> I'd always said to myself, I'm not going to do it if it's the wrong time, you know, I'm not going to do it when I don't want to. I'll just

---

35. Sharon Thompson, *Going All the Way: Teenage Girls' Tales of Sex, Romance, and Pregnancy* (New York: Hill and Wang, 1995), 249. Thompson points out that Anja's ability to see the humor in this situation reflects confidence and maturity. Narrators who could tell a funny story had a firm sense of self.

wait till I really want to. And I did want to and I was glad I wanted to and you know, that moment was right.[36]

This voice belongs to a girl with a much more mature approach to sex than many of her peers. Anja felt good about her decision to have sex with Monty: she really liked him, she was sexually attracted to him, and she thought the timing was right. She even admits to a certain amount of cool calculation — "it was another thing I could get out of the way" — perhaps an attempt to maintain distance or maybe evidence that for Anja, first sex was just first sex: something worth waiting for but not an earth-shattering milestone.

Sharon Thompson argues that girls who can name their desire and put it in the right perspective (she calls them "pleasure narrators") can do so because they grew up around other people who could. One of her interviewees, Annie, described the connection between her childhood and her attitude during adolescence about sexual activity: "I wasn't really that shy because I had grown up around it [sex] and it seemed sort of natural to me." Eloida remembered conversations among older women in which she had been included:

We were just sitting listening to older women talking about sex, you know, sometimes in very intricate details, sometimes, you know, just jokes about it. Also, you know, problems with men — like, you know, "Oh god, stood up again. Those jazz musicians always stand us up. . . . Next time I'm going to get a man with a car and a job."

Jen reported that her mother "had always talked very casually about sex." She described for Thompson those conversations with her mother, emphasizing how light-hearted and even mundane they were:

I mean, I have sat at the dinner table and discussed with mom what contraceptive she used when she was, uh, uh, you know, having an affair with my dad for the year before she married him. And, uhm, actually we have discussed what sex was like with my father and what she did in — in the way of fooling around before she got married. She told me all these wonderful incidents about the back seat of the car, which I thought was hysterical. I can't imagine anybody bothering to use the back seat of a car. Yeah, and we once

---

36. *Going All the Way,* 278.

over dinner talked about pregnancy and giving birth. Sitting in a restaurant. While we ate.[37]

Girls who go into erotic relationships with a stance of friendly distrust generally survive them unscathed because they have maintained a limited and realistic sense of the future possibilities, which doesn't necessarily mean that they experience no pain when relationships end. Anja recalls her breakup with Monty by saying, "And I sort of felt like, Oh no, because I really did like him."[38] Compare this, however, to Tracy from chapter 4: "No one's ever going to hurt me that way again and I'll make sure of it. . . . My idea right now is that I don't think I'm ever going to let a guy touch me again until I'm engaged or married."[39] Friendly distrust allows girls to keep a level-headed view about their relationships. They may not know for sure what erotic involvement means in the end, but they adopt a healthy skepticism that keeps them safe. One girl described to Thompson her attitude toward the dissolution of a relationship by saying, in effect, that she refused to let it dominate her view of all romance: "At that point, it was a lot easier to decide that I hated him than that I hated most men, so I decided the guy was a real schmo. Well, interesting experience."[40] Friendly distrust also allows girls to try new relationships in the future: "If you have one guy who likes you, it gives you the confidence to like another guy and be successful at it."[41]

In most cases the preferred approach for adolescent sexual relationships would be ones of friendly distrust. Analyzing them as relationships of trust has given us another important way of seeing what is wrong with so many adolescent sexual relationships. They are wrong not because sexual activity is dangerous for teenagers, although it can be; nor because adolescents are too immature to be sexually involved, though this assertion may be true. Rather, adolescent relationships are too often disingenuous and sometimes even coercive, which by no means indicates that all adolescent boys are manipulators and all adolescent girls dupes. The

---

37. Sharon Thompson, "Putting a Big Thing into a Little Hole: Teenage Girls' Accounts of Sexual Initiation," in *Journal of Sex Research* 27, no. 3 (August 1990): 354–55. Thompson summarizes: "Through these conversations, these daughters gain invaluable insights into the body and intimate relations, and they learn that talking about their pleasures, sorrows, and furies will strengthen, inform, and enrich their lives" (354).

38. *Going All the Way*, 280.
39. *Going All the Way*, 43.
40. *Going All the Way*, 274.
41. *Going All the Way*, 274.

real issue at stake in the morality of a trust relationship, we recall, is the extent of unwarranted reliance on the other. As Baier (cited previously) argues, "a trust relationship is morally bad *to the extent that* either party relies on qualities in the other which would be weakened by the knowledge that the other relies on them." Many if not most people likely rely on qualities in their romantic partners that are at times unrealistic and even mildly coercive; indeed, part of desiring someone erotically are the fantasies and idealizations that accompany ordinary attraction. But the problem is that adolescent girls too often place too much unacknowledged trust in their partners, in part because they are still trying to solve the problem of needing to trust in others while being independent selves, and they solve the problem wrong. They enter relationships that can only be sustained through artifice of some kind, whether it is self-deception or self-disavowal or simply pretending.

Distrust within sexual relationships, on the other hand, would protect girls while they journey through the psychic struggles of adolescence. They would be free to admit their distress because the stakes would be lower. They would construct sexual relationship as something enjoyable and meaningful but no guarantee of lasting happiness. They would be empowered to ask for what they want and demand, at the very least, honesty of their partners.

Why do I advocate distrust rather than some other moral norm? Sexual ethics has long relied on related concepts like love, honesty, and consent to provide the standards for the time to engage in sexual activity. Without claiming that the appropriate level of trust provides the only moral standard we need, we can identify certain advantages to it over these other concepts. Love alone does not ensure safety and, as we have seen, love can be seriously misconstrued. Honesty is very important, but it can be brutal or ineffective. Some sexual ethicists advocate mutual consent, but this status can too easily degenerate into silent consent to what another wants. Feminist theologians of the erotic talk a great deal about relationality; but as we have already seen, being relational is no guarantor of improper invulnerability, and fanning that flame may sometimes even become dangerous. Trust is the most precise term for the norm we seek when we have identified vulnerability and ambiguity as the primary moral challenges. When people can trust one another in relationship — or, alternatively, when friendly distrust is sustained — they enjoy some degree of protection despite their vulnerability.

SEVEN

After Feminist Theologies
of the Erotic

W E ARE NOW IN A POSITION to return to our analysis of the
feminist theologians of the erotic with which this book began.
As I have shown, we need to change some of what feminist theologians
of the erotic have done for the sake of achieving a viable sexual ethic.
We need to make more modest and practical claims about the way we
value and evaluate erotic experience. My aim, unlike theirs, has not been
to "recover" Eros, for I do not think such a project finally makes sense,
but to move beyond our attempts to stipulate its meaning.

I suggest instead a healthy skepticism regarding the relationship between morality and the erotic. Feminist theologians of the erotic, as I
argued in detail in chapter 2, wish to elevate the status of the erotic and
place it on par with Agape as an exemplary form of human love. They
would reverse the Christian tradition's devaluation of erotic passions and
feelings, suggesting instead that expressions of erotic passion represent the
true fulfillment of Christian love. This reversal is necessary, they argue,
because people's failure to flourish and love rightly results from a dearth of
Eros. Too many people misunderstand and abuse erotic passion and thus
invite misery and injustice, sometimes even upon themselves. People are
unaware that Eros is the key to a good life. Contrary to popular perception,
according to these theologians, Eros has the power to usher in genuinely
loving relationships between people, not only on the interpersonal level,
but even in community.

Theologically, feminist theologians of the erotic have aimed to subvert
traditional (patriarchal) theology and insert in its stead a feminist version
of Eros, which is positive and even glowing. They place a feminist erotic
where an androcentric, patriarchal erotic once stood. Writing about this
tendency among feminist theologians, Kathleen Sands asserts:

In fact, what patriarchal religion had demonized or inferiorized is now identified with the divine or taken as a privileged conduit of divine revelation. . . . The feminist good — be it "Eros," "nature," or "women's experience" — is often justified in the face of its apparent moral failures, and the ultimate power of this good is asserted over the apparent victory of patriarchy.[1]

Feminist theologians of the erotic tend to ignore its moral ambiguities and instead assert its power and supremacy as a moral good in human life. The erotic becomes "the feminist good" in these theologies.

One result of this theological strategy, especially relevant to human sexual life, is that the erotic ends up providing its own moral justification, which leaves little room for justification for or judgment of erotic relationships. Claiming that the power of the erotic erases any moral failures *of* the erotic is saying that the erotic justifies and judges itself. This claim represents a faulty way of relating morality to Eros.[2]

The evidence and theory supplied in chapters 4 and 5 suggest that erotic relationships need moral guidance. These chapters examined in detail how adolescent girls actually experience erotic relationship and found that for them the erotic is not an unambiguous good. Adolescents' erotic narratives clearly suggest that many girls are wiser than to think that erotic experience necessarily provides the key to a good life, whether they construe that as romance, intimacy, physical passion, or something else altogether. Too often, girls' erotic passion spells trouble for them, and not solely or even primarily because their passion is not genuine. Drawn erotically into sexual relationship by the promise of romance, for example, many of them are hurt by their own intense yearning to love and be loved by their boyfriends. Despite how deeply and genuinely it may be felt, that yearning ultimately traps rather than liberates them, at least within the social context of contemporary adolescence where girls still frequently enjoy less power than boys to realize their passion. This example is just one of how, in practice, the erotic is not always particularly powerful or liberating.

---

1. Kathleen Sands, "Uses of the Thea(o)logian: Sex and Theodicy in Religious Feminism," *Journal for the Feminist Study of Religion* 8 (spring 1992): 8–9.

2. This remains true even if the erotic is primarily constructed as love, which presumably needs little justification. Ethicists increasingly recognize that even love has moral limits — that it is possible to love "too much" or too unconditionally. Even Agape needs to be fenced in, or at least balanced, by other centers of value in the moral life. Love itself, in other words, requires moral boundaries, like self-respect, justice, and reciprocity, to temper and shape it.

The theories employed in chapter 5 explain why. We learned that individuals take their meaning for erotic experience in large part from early familial relationships. Its meanings are largely molded in the forge of gendered family dynamics. That which people find erotically compelling is deeply tied to the wider relations of power that occur between mothers and fathers and men and women more generally. The meaning of the erotic is therefore inescapably constructed at a psychic level out of social and cultural relations of power. No untouched, morally pure Eros can free people from their experiences.

Therefore, rather than celebrating the moral value of the erotic, people need practical moral guidelines that take into account the constructed character of the erotic into account. Individuals need safety and some way of reducing their vulnerability within relationships that encompass differences in power. Erotic relationships, unreliable as they are to assuring our flourishing, and even notorious for disempowering us, call for norms that will protect us when we are nevertheless drawn into them. Chapter 6 therefore framed erotic relationships as trust relationships. According to this perspective, while sexual relationships may not ensure the good life, they should at the very least not render partners *more* vulnerable to the vagary and instability of erotic passion. This approach does not presume erotic relationships between individuals to be naturally or essentially trustworthy, as some feminist theologies of the erotic imply. An ethic of trust is superior to an ethic of erotic liberation for these reasons and should form the basis of our sexual ethics.

While based upon philosophical rather than theological ideas about trust, and informed by sources such as social history and psychoanalytic theory, a sexual ethic of trust such as I have outlined fits into a larger theological ethic of sexuality in at least the following ways. First, this ethic ultimately serves a theological ethic insofar as it provides an important part of what would follow from a sexual ethic that ultimately rests on theological beliefs about embodied life and its passions. This ethic and this book are grounded in an implicit incarnational theology, that is, a theology of the body that affirms the finitude, historicity, limitation, but also sacrality of embodied human life. Admittedly, this kind of "body theology" is itself still a work in progress; indeed, theologies of the body are relatively new.[3] But their roots

---

3. See Lisa Isherwood and Elizabeth Stuart, *Introducing Body Theology* (Cleveland: Pilgrim Press, 1998).

can be traced within both Catholic and Protestant tradition. According to the incarnational perspective I take, which recognizes the moral ambiguity of embodied life, that we should heap any more praise on our sensuality and embodiment even while we have no reason to despise, deny, or minimize them either is far from clear.[4] Our bodies are a significant part of our created nature as humans, and our created nature is a gift and a greatly good thing.

Second, a Christian feminist theological ethic of sexuality arising from this study would blend skepticism about human sexual life and hope for its transformation in equal measure, based not only upon evidence derived from the work of social scientists and theorists, but also on a strong view of sin derived from Protestant tradition. Implicit throughout the present work has been the assumption that we sin as sexual beings — not perhaps more than we sin in other ways — but we are at least sinful as sexual beings. Yet we are also saved from sin by grace. The potential for sexual sin, in other words, can never be ignored, as Augustine and Luther and Calvin knew. In particular, sin, sexuality, and the human capacity to create meaning are deeply intertwined. As humans, we are endowed with the ability and given the freedom to construct all manner of meanings for our sexuality, but whether this freedom is a gift is finally ambiguous. Our freedom is literally a mixed blessing. In the end, sometimes we are able to transform the meanings of sexuality we create and sometimes we are not. When we are not able, we fall back on the grace of God, which is ultimately the only transformative power. In God's grace lies the hope for making all things new.

More remains to be done to locate this project securely within a larger theological ethic. Its ties to Christian theological tradition would need to be made more explicit, which would involve a chastened retrieval of tradition, especially following streams within Protestant thought. Another task would be to discern the scriptural witness that grounds the particular convictions elaborated herein. Finally, we would need to trace the ways that the Christian community has sought to be the body of Christ by embodying together a passionate and trusting love.

---

4. Like sexual ethicists, medical ethicists who identify with a theological tradition struggle to determine the right way to value life lived within the limits of the human body. In medical ethics, perhaps even more than sexual ethics, the dilemma revolves around the age-old question of whether we *have* or *are* our bodies. In other words, ought we to transcend the limitations of our embodiment when we have the technological and medical means to do so, or ought we accept and accede to them? See, for example, Gilbert Meilaender, "How Bioethics Lost the Body: Personhood," in *Body, Soul, and Bioethics* (Notre Dame, Ind.: University of Notre Dame Press, 1995), and *Embodiment, Morality, and Medicine*, ed. Lisa Sowle Cahill and Margaret A. Farley (Boston: Kluwer Academic Publishers, 1995).

Works Cited

American Association of University Women. *Shortchanging Girls, Shortchanging America: Full Data Report.* Washington, D.C.: American Association of University Women, 1990.

Andolsen, Barbara Hilkert. "Whose Sexuality? Whose Tradition? Women, Experience, and Roman Catholic Sexual Ethics." In *Religion and Sexual Health,* edited by Ronald M. Green, 55–77. Boston: Kluwer Academic Publishers, 1992.

Aquinas, Thomas. *Summa Theologica.* In *Introduction to St. Thomas Aquinas,* edited by Anton C. Pegis. The Modern Library. New York: Random House, 1945.

Augustine. *Confessions.* Translated by R. S. Pine-Coffin. London: Penguin Books, 1961.

———. *City of God.* Edited by Vernon J. Bourke. Image Books. Garden City, N.Y.: Doubleday & Company, 1958.

Baier, Annette C. *Moral Prejudices: Essays on Ethics.* Cambridge: Harvard University Press, 1994.

Bartky, Sandra. "Feminine Masochism and the Politics of Personal Transformation." In *Philosophy of Sex: Contemporary Readings.* 2d ed., edited by Alan Soble, 219–42. Savage, Md.: Rowman and Littlefield, 1991.

Benhabib, Seyla. *Situating the Self: Gender, Community and Postmodernism in Contemporary Ethics.* New York: Routledge, 1992.

Benjamin, Jessica. *Bonds of Love: Psychoanalysis, Feminism, and the Problem of Domination.* New York: Pantheon Books, 1988.

Brock, Rita Nakashima. *Journeys by Heart: A Christology of Erotic Power.* New York: Crossroad, 1988.

Brown, Lyn Mikel, and Carol Gilligan. *Meeting at the Crossroads: Women's Psychology and Girls' Development.* Cambridge: Harvard University Press, 1992.

Burnaby, John. "Love: Historical Perspectives." In *The Westminster Dictionary of Christian Ethics,* edited by James F. Childress and John Macquarrie. Philadelphia: Westminster Press, 1986.

Cahill, Lisa, and Margaret A. Farley, eds. *Embodiment, Morality, and Medicine.* Boston: Kluwer Academic Publishers, 1995.

Cahill, Lisa Sowle, and James F. Childress. *Christian Ethics: Problems and Prospects.* Cleveland: Pilgrim Press, 1996.

Chasseguet-Smirgel, Janine, ed. *Female Sexuality.* Ann Arbor: University of Michigan Press, 1970.

Chodorow, Nancy. *Femininities, Masculinities, Sexualities: Freud and Beyond.* Lexington: University Press of Kentucky, 1994.

———. *The Reproduction of Mothering: Psychoanalysis and the Sociology of Gender.* Berkeley: University of California Press, 1978.

Chopp, Rebecca. "Seeing and Naming the World Anew: The Works of Rosemary Radford Ruether." *Religious Studies Review* 15, no. 1 (January 1989): 1–11.

———. "Feminism's Theological Pragmatics: A Social Naturalism of Women's Experience." *Journal of Religion* 67, no. 2 (April 1987): 239–56.

Chopp, Rebecca, and Sheila Greeve Davaney, eds. *Horizons in Feminist Theology: Identity, Tradition, and Norms.* Minneapolis: Fortress Press, 1997.

Clark, J. Michael. *A Defiant Celebration: Theological Ethics and Gay Sexuality.* Garland, Tex.: Tangelwuld, 1990.

Cooey, Paula, Sharon Farmer, and Mary Ellen Ross, eds. *Embodied Love: Sensuality and Relationship as Feminist Values.* San Francisco: Harper & Row, 1988.

Deutsch, Helene. *Psychology of Women.* Vol. 1. New York: Grune & Stratton, 1944.

Ellison, Marvin. *Erotic Justice: A Liberating Ethic of Sexuality.* Louisville: Westminster/John Knox Press, 1996.

Farley, Margaret. *Just Love: Sexual Ethics and Social Change.* New York: Crossroad, 1998.

Farley, Margaret A. *Personal Commitments: Beginning, Keeping, Changing.* San Francisco: Harper & Row Publishers, 1986.

Flax, Jane. *Thinking Fragments: Psychoanalysis, Feminism, and Postmodernism in the Contemporary West.* Berkeley: University of California Press, 1990.

Foucault, Michel. *The History of Sexuality, Volume 1: An Introduction.* New York: Random House, 1978.

———. "Truth and Power." In *Power/Knowledge: Selected Interviews and Other Writings,* edited by Colin Gordon. New York: Pantheon, 1980.

Freud, Sigmund. "The Ego and the Id." In *The Standard Edition of the Complete Psychological Works.* London: The Hogarth Press, 1923/1957.

Fulkerson, Mary McClintock. *Changing the Subject: Women's Discourses and Feminist Theology.* Minneapolis: Fortress Press, 1994.

Gagnon, John H., and William Simon, eds. *The Sexual Scene.* Chicago: Aldine Publishing Company, 1970.

Gilligan, Carol. *In a Different Voice: Psychological Theory and Women's Development.* Cambridge: Harvard University Press, 1982.

Gilson, Anne Bathurst. *Eros Breaking Free: Interpreting Sexual Theo-Ethics.* Cleveland: Pilgrim Press, 1995.

Goldstein, Valerie Saiving. "The Human Situation: A Feminine View." *Journal of Religion* 40 (1960): 100–112.

Grant, Colin. "For the Love of God." *Journal of Religious Ethics* 24, no. 1 (spring 1996).

Hersch, Patricia. *A Tribe Apart: A Journey into the Heart of American Adolescence.* New York: Ballantine Books, 1998.

Heyward, Carter. "Lamenting the Loss of Love." *Journal of Religious Ethics* 24, no. 1 (spring 1996).

———. *Our Passion for Justice: Images of Power, Sexuality, and Liberation.* New York: Pilgrim Press, 1984.

———. *The Redemption of God: A Theology of Mutual Relation.* Lanham, Md.: University Press of America, 1982.

————. *Touching Our Strength: The Erotic as Power and the Love of God.* San Francisco: HarperSanFrancisco, 1989.

hooks, bell. *Feminist Theory: From Margin to Center.* Boston: South End Press, 1984.

Horney, Karen. "The Flight from Womanhood: The Masculinity Complex in Women as Viewed by Men and Women." *International Journal of Psychoanalysis* 7 (1926): 324–39.

Irwin, Alexander C. *Eros toward the World: Paul Tillich and the Theology of the Erotic.* Minneapolis: Fortress Press, 1991.

Isasi-Díaz, Ada María. "Experiences." In *Dictionary of Feminist Theologies,* edited by Letty M. Russell and J. Shannon Clarkson, 95–96. Louisville, Ky.: Westminster/John Knox Press, 1996.

Isherwood, Lisa, and Elizabeth Stuart. *Introducing Body Theology.* Cleveland: Pilgrim Press, 1998.

Jonte-Pace, Diana. "Psychoanalysis after Feminism." *Religious Studies Review* 19, no. 2 (April 1993): 110–15.

Jordan, Judith. "Empathy and the Mother-Daughter Relationship." *Work in Progress* no. 82–02. Wellesley, Mass.: The Stone Center Working Paper Series, 1983.

Keller, Jean. "Autonomy, Relationality, and Feminist Ethics." *Hypatia* 12, no. 2 (spring 1997): 152–64.

Kittay, Eva Feder, and Diana T. Meyers, eds. *Women and Moral Theory.* Totowa, N.J.: Rowman and Littlefield, 1987.

Lawson, Annette and Deborah L. Rhode, eds. *The Politics of Pregnancy: Adolescent Sexuality and Public Policy.* New Haven: Yale University Press, 1993.

Lorde, Audre. *Sister Outsider: Essays and Speeches by Audre Lorde.* Trumansburg, N.Y.: Crossing Press, 1984.

Luban, David. *The Good Lawyer: Lawyers' Roles and Lawyers' Ethics.* Totowa, N.J.: Rowman and Allanheld, 1984.

Luhmann, Niklas. *Trust and Power.* New York: John Wiley & Sons, 1979.

MacKinnon, Catharine. *Toward a Feminist Theory of the State.* Cambridge: Harvard University Press, 1989.

Mahler, Margaret, Fred Pine, and Anni Bergmann. *The Psychological Birth of the Human Infant.* New York: Basic Books, 1975.

May, William F. "Professional Ethics: Setting, Terrain, and Teacher." In *Ethics Teaching in Higher Education,* edited by Daniel Callahan and Sissela Bok. New York: Plenum, 1980.

————. *The Physician's Covenant: Images of the Healer in Medical Ethics.* Philadelphia: Westminster Press, 1983.

Meilaender, Gilbert. "How Bioethics Lost the Body: Personhood." *Body, Soul, and Bioethics.* Notre Dame, Ind.: University of Notre Dame Press, 1995.

————. *Letters to Ellen.* Grand Rapids: William B. Eerdmans Publishing Co., 1996.

Miller, Jean Baker. "What Do We Mean by Relationship?" *Work in Progress* no. 22. Wellesley, Mass.: The Stone Center Working Paper Series, 1986.

Moore, Susan, and Doreen Rosenthal. "The Social Context of Adolescent Sexuality: Safe Sex Implications." *Journal of Adolescence* 15 (1992).

Nagel, Thomas. *Mortal Questions.* Cambridge: Cambridge University Press, 1979.

Nelson, James. *Between Two Gardens: Reflections on Sexuality and Religious Experience.* Cleveland: Pilgrim Press, 1983.

———. *Body Theology.* Louisville, Ky.: Westminster/John Knox Press, 1992.

———. *Embodiment: An Approach to Sexuality and Christian Theology.* Minneapolis: Augsburg Publishing House, 1978.

———. *The Intimate Connection: Male Sexuality, Masculine Spirituality.* Philadelphia: Westminster Press, 1988.

Nelson, James, and Sandra Longfellow, eds. *Sexuality and the Sacred: Sources for Theological Reflection.* Louisville, Ky.: Westminster/John Knox Press, 1994.

Nygren, Anders. *Agape and Eros.* Translated by Philip Watson. Philadelphia: Westminster Press, 1953.

Orenstein, Peggy. *SchoolGirls: Young Women, Self-Esteem, and the Confidence Gap.* New York: Bantam Doubleday Dell Publishing Group, 1994.

Outka, Gene. "Love." In *Encyclopedia of Ethics,* edited by Lawrence C. Becker and Charlotte Becker, 742–51. New York: Garland Publications, 1992.

Pellegrino, Edmund D., Robert M. Veatch, and John P. Langan, eds. *Ethics, Trust and the Professions: Philosophical and Cultural Aspects.* Washington, D.C.: Georgetown University Press, 1991.

Phillips, Lynn, ed. *The Girls Report: What We Know and Need to Know about Growing Up Female.* New York: National Council for Research on Women, 1998.

Plaskow, Judith. *Sex, Sin and Grace: Women's Experience and the Theologies of Reinhold Niebuhr and Paul Tillich.* Washington, D.C.: University Press of America, 1980.

———. *Standing Again at Sinai: Judaism from a Feminist Perspective.* San Francisco: Harper Collins, 1990.

Plaskow, Judith, and Carol P. Christ, eds. *Weaving the Visions: New Patterns in Feminist Spirituality.* San Francisco: HarperSanFrancisco, 1989.

Plato. *The Symposium.* In *Plato's Erotic Dialogues,* translated by William S. Cobb. Albany: State University of New York Press, 1993.

Russell, Letty M. *Feminist Interpretation of the Bible.* Philadelphia: Westminster Press, 1985.

Sands, Kathleen. "Uses of the Thea(o)logian: Sex and Theodicy in Religious Feminism." *Journal for the Feminist Study of Religion* 8 (spring 1992): 7–33.

Sedgwick, Timothy. Paper delivered at the Society of Christian Ethics Annual Meeting, February 1993.

Singer, Irving. *The Nature of Love.* Vol. 1. Chicago: University of Chicago Press, 1984.

Snitow, Ann Barr, Christine Stansell, and Sharon Thompson, eds. *Powers of Desire: The Politics of Sexuality.* New York: Monthly Review Press, 1983.

Stern, Daniel. *The Interpersonal World of the Infant: A View from Psychoanalysis and Developmental Psychology.* New York: Basic Books, 1985.

Stern, Lori. "Disavowing the Self in Female Adolescence." *Women and Therapy* 2, no. 3–4 (1991): 105–17.

Surrey, Janet L. "Relationship and Empowerment." *Work in Progress* no. 30. Wellesley, Mass.: The Stone Center Working Paper Series, 1983.

Tanenbaum, Leora. *Slut! Growing Up Female with a Bad Reputation.* New York: Seven Stories Press, 1999.

Thompson, Clara. "Cultural Pressures in the Psychology of Women." *Psychiatry* 5, no. 3 (August 1942): 331–39.

Thompson, Sharon. *Going All the Way: Teenage Girls' Tales of Sex, Romance, and Pregnancy.* New York: Hill and Wang, 1995.

———. "Putting a Big Thing into a Little Hole: Teenage Girls' Accounts of Sexual Initiation." *Journal of Sex Research* 27, no. 3 (August 1990): 341–61.

———. "Search for Tomorrow: Feminism and the Reconstruction of Teen Romance." In *Pleasure and Danger: Exploring Female Sexuality,* edited by Carole S. Vance. London: Routledge and Kegan Paul, 1984.

Uhrig, Larry J. *Sex Positive: A Gay Contribution to Sexual and Spiritual Union.* Boston: Alyson Publications, 1986.

Vacek, Edward. "Love: Christian and Diverse." *Journal of Religious Ethics* 24, no. 1 (spring 1996).

Vance, Carole, ed. *Pleasure and Danger: Exploring Female Sexuality.* London: Routledge and Kegan Paul, 1984.

Vinovskis, Maris A. "An 'Epidemic' of Adolescent Pregnancy? Some Historical Considerations." *Journal of Family History* 6, no. 2 (summer 1981).

Wallwork, Ernest. *Psychoanalysis and Ethics.* New Haven: Yale University Press, 1991.

Webster, Alison R. *Found Wanting: Women, Christianity, and Sexuality.* London: Cassell, 1995.

Weeks, Jeffrey. *Sexuality and Its Discontents.* London: Routledge & Kegan Paul, 1985.

Williams, Bernard. "Politics and Moral Character." In *Public and Private Morality,* edited by Stuart Hampshire. New York: Cambridge University Press, 1978.

Winter, Laraine. "The Role of Sexual Self-Concept in the Use of Contraceptives." *Family Planning Perspectives* 20 (1988): 123–27.

Zabin, Laurie Schwab, and Samuel D. Clark. "Why They Delay." *Family Planning Perspectives* 13 (1981): 205–17.

Index

self
  disavowal of. *See* disavowal of self
  sense of, 45, 50, 68, 97, 100,
    126–31, 137–39, 143, 145–46,
    149
  theories of, 14, 33n
separation, 119, 137–42, 145–46
sensuality. *See* erotic as sensuality
sex-negativity, 13, 26, 53, 56
sex-positivity, 13, 27–28, 56–57,
  67–68
sexual ethics, 5–8, 9, 12n, 17–18, 42,
  51–52, 59, 69–70, 83, 188–89
Simon, William, 54
social constructionism, 2–3, 54–56,
  63–66, 114, 136
Sokolowski, Robert, 174
Stern, Lori, 119, 127–32, 179

Tanenbaum, Leora, 92, 95
theory, need for, 9, 53, 54, 117–18,
  153–58
Thompson, Clara, 128
Thompson, Sharon, 3, 7–8, 89–90,
  103, 104, 106, 107, 112, 113,
  180

trust
  adolescent sexuality and, 180–86
  justification for, 166–71
  nature of, 162–66
  professional-client, 172–77
truth, 1, 10, 40, 46–47, 78–80,
  85–86n

universalism, 41–42

Veatch, Robert, 172, 175–76, 177
voice, loss of
  demonstrated, 121–24
  theorized, 88, 124–26
vulnerability, 97–98, 111–13, 166–69,
  172–74, 181–82

Weeks, Jeffrey, 60, 83
Western tradition, 21, 23, 24, 31, 37
wisdom. *See* erotic as wisdom
women's experience, 70–72
  commonality of, 72–76, 156
  divinity of, 81–82, 158
  normativeness of, 76–81, 157

Zaner, Richard, 173